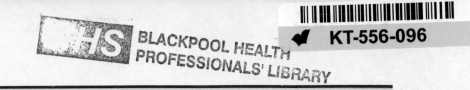 ✔ KT-556-096

Clinical Audit

Edited by

Irene Higginson

Senior Lecturer/Consultant, Health Services Research Unit,
London School of Hygiene and Tropical Medicine

With a Foreword by

Geoffrey W Hanks

Professor of Palliative Medicine
University of Bristol

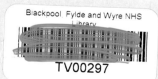
RADCLIFFE   YORK

©1993 Radcliffe Medical Press Ltd
18 Marcham Road, Abingdon, Oxon, OX14 1AA, UK

Radcliffe Medical Press, Inc.
141 Fifth Avenue, New York, NY 10010, USA

Reprinted 1995

British Library Cataloguing in Publication Data

A catalogue record for this book is available from the British Library.

1 870905 64 4

Typeset by Advance Typesetting Ltd, Oxfordshire
Printed and bound in Great Britain

Contents

Foreword

Audit has only recently become part of the language of medicine, yet in a short period of time it has become a day to day feature of clinical practice. Audit has brought with it some new jargon and in recent years has spawned committees, officers, computer software, books, journals and of course meetings. To what end? The aim is clear enough: the objective of clinical audit is to improve the quality of care provided for patients by doctors and other health care workers. What is not yet so clear is how best to implement audit in different clinical settings or how effective are the methods of audit currently in use.

The focus on quality is not a domestic or local issue or confined to any particular specialty. The World Health Organization suggested that 'by 1990, all member states should have built effective mechanisms for ensuring the quality of patient care'. In the UK the Government White Paper *Working for Patients* required that every health district must have in place by 1991 some system of medical audit. In such a climate it is unsurprising to find a text on clinical audit in palliative care, although on the face of it this is a particularly difficult area to measure and evaluate.

It may be a surprise to many to learn that clinical standard setting and the evaluation of care was recognized as essential to the development of palliative care from its beginnings in the 1960s, and this has perhaps given us a headstart now. In an early study at St Christopher's Hospice, surviving spouses of patients who had died of cancer in the hospice or in local hospitals were asked about the care patients had received. This approach implicitly recognized that traditional outcome measures of morbidity and mortality were not applicable. Subjective assessment by 'consumers' of health care is now generally adopted as an audit measure in other areas of clinical practice.

There has been much activity recently in palliative care services to set standards of care and to produce guidelines of 'best practice'. Palliative care is multidisciplinary care and is highly dependent on effective team working. The focus of care is not the patient in isolation, but the patient and his or her family. Thus clinical audit in palliative care must be multidisciplinary and outcome measures must encompass not just the patient but those around him. This causes particular difficulties for the would-be clinical auditor, and this book will provide much practical advice to guide him or her towards some solutions.

Irene Higginson has put together a comprehensive review of clinical audit in palliative care. She has drawn from her extensive personal experience in developing audit tools for palliative care and has brought together contributions from others who have direct experience of audit both within and outside the specialty.

Clinical audit is here to stay and this means that everyone involved in health care delivery, including those of us in palliative care must know about it, understand it and do it. In the UK audit is now an invariable feature of contracts between purchasers and providers, although it would be naive to believe that at present contracting for clinical quality is the norm. However, the aim of clinical audit is not just to satisfy current exigencies of health care delivery imposed by government. The aim is to improve the care of patients, and I have no doubt that this book will help those working in palliative care to achieve that.

GEOFFREY W HANKS
August 1993

Contributors

Julia Addington-Hall
Department of Epidemiology and Public Health, University College, London

Eduardo Bruera
Director, Palliative Care Program, Edmonton General Hospital, Edmonton, Canada

Elizabeth Butters
Health Services Research Unit, London School of Hygiene and Tropical Medicine, London

Robert A Catterall
Medical Director, St Barnabas' Hospice, Lincoln

Janet Doyle
Regional Nurse – Continuing Care, East Anglian Regional Health Authority, Cambridge

Ilora Finlay
Consultant Medical Director, Holme Tower Marie Curie Centre, Penarth, South Glamorgan

Robert George
Consultant in Palliative Medicine, Palliative Care Team, Camden and Islington Community Health Services NHS Trust, London

Geoffrey W Hanks
Professor of Palliative Medicine, University of Bristol

Anne Hayes
Nurse Tutor, Our Lady's Hospice, Dublin, Eire

Irene Higginson
Senior Lecturer/Consultant, Health Services Research Unit,
London School of Hygiene and Tropical Medicine, London

Anthony Hopkins
Director, Research Unit, Royal College of Physicians, London

John Hunt
Senior Nurse, Nightingale Macmillan Continuing Care Unit, Derby

Susan MacDonald
Palliative Care Program, Edmonton General Hospital, Edmonton,
Canada

Mark McCarthy
Department of Epidemiology and Public Health, University College,
London

Maura McDonnell
Palliative Care Co-ordinator, Irish Cancer Society, Dublin, Eire

Elizabeth McKee
Assistant Nursing Director (Home Care), Northern Ireland Hospice,
Belfast

Finbarr Murphy
Irish Cancer Society, Dublin, Eire

Charles D Shaw
Director, Bristol Clinical Audit Unit, Department of Epidemiology
and Public Health Medicine, University of Bristol, Bristol

Introduction to Audit in Palliative Care

CHARLES D SHAW

Quality in health care

Concern for quality in health care has long been explicit in the market-oriented environment of the United States and Canada where it has been partially driven by risk management and cost containment. In the United Kingdom, until recently, it has been relatively implicit and driven by clinical concerns for professional self-regulation although the pursuit of management control has been promoted by the purchaser/provider split. Throughout the world there has been a growing concern for value for money in health care which cannot be resolved by increasing national expenditure. Although each country differs in its organization and funding of health care the general principles of quality management apply universally.

Development in the United Kingdom National Health Service

A number of national reports had argued the case for active and regular review of the performance of the Health Service and of its staff during the 1970s. These included the Cogwheels Report[1], the Briggs Report[2] on nursing and the Alment Report[3]. The Royal Commission said 'we are not convinced that the professions generally regard the introduction of audit or peer review of standards of care and treatment with a proper sense of urgency[4].'

In 1983, the Griffiths Report on management of the National Health Service[5], recommended the appointment of senior officers to direct the growth of quality assurance in the service. Since many of these directors of quality appointed during the late 1980s were formerly nursing officers, particular attention was given to customer service and in the professional sphere to nursing. In the next few years attention turned to competitive tendering for support services such as catering, domestic and transport, which forced managers and providers of service to identify and measure acceptable levels not only of cost and quantity but also of quality in these areas.

However, attention finally turned to medical practice in the White Paper, *Working for Patients*[6], and the subsequent working papers on medical audit. These define medical audit as 'the systematic, critical analysis of the quality of medical care including the procedures used for diagnosis and treatment, the use of resources and the resulting outcome and quality of life for the patient'. This formal recognition of the principle of medical audit and the commitment of funding to support it was generally well received by the medical profession as a mechanism for professional education and training. However, it was also welcomed by managers as a potential mechanism for accountability and control – particularly with reference to the forthcoming purchaser/provider split which would require close monitoring of clinical performance in contracts.

Approaches to quality in the NHS

Audit is but one part of the broader concept of quality management; from the viewpoint of health service management, this may be approached by three routes:

- *direct:* managers can take direct action to provide a framework for total quality through definition of standards, information, resources and mechanisms for effecting change in the organization
- *external:* managers can also heed review by legitimate outside bodies such as statutory inspectorates, the national professional training bodies and community health councils. There has been little co-ordination between these various groups and often their reports were not available to the managers concerned. Indeed the failure of these bodies to provide coherent standards, monitoring or follow-up in the past, combined with the prospect of more independent and competitive health care providers, argues strongly for an independent national co-ordination of the accreditation function
- *indirect:* ultimately all managers must provide for and rely upon the internal review of technical quality of clinical practice by the professional groups themselves. This includes medical, paramedical, nursing or, in combination, 'clinical' audit.

Audit and clinical quality assurance

The purpose of audit generally agreed among the medical professional bodies is first the improvement of care to individual patients, second the education and training of individual clinicians and third the effective use of resources. This does not equate to purchasing of computers (even though they may be helpful in processing and presenting data); it is not the same as medical research (research seeks to identify best practice; audit seeks to ask whether that is being applied locally); it is not resource management (although it shares an urgent need to define numerically the clinical workload, clinical practice and clinical outcomes).

One way to consider health services is to see them as a production line generating 'health' from a defined set of resources or inputs. This has four main elements:

- inputs: resources in terms of manpower, equipment and money, a traditional and relatively easily quantified measure
- process: how the resources are organized such as in counselling, prescribing and domiciliary visits
- output: productivity or throughput such as clinic attendance rate, discharge rate
- outcome: achievement of intended results.

Even if these four elements can be measured, the relationship between them is variable and ill-defined, the quality of care is hard to quantify, and in many conditions the ideal outcome is not agreed. Although results are ultimately the criteria by which any service should be judged, the outcome of health care is, in practice, often difficult or impossible to measure. For this reason, some authors prefer to focus on selected 'intermediate' outcomes which can be more readily related to the care given. In many circumstances, however, a quicker and simpler assessment of care is based upon the examination of process, for example, what was done to the patient. Justification for this approach relies heavily on evidence that what is assumed to be a good process will produce a good outcome. Ideally this will be based on evidence from clinical trials, but frequently there is little more than anecdotal evidence for the effectiveness of clinical processes.

Effective audit may be seen as a cyclical activity with three principal stages, the first stage is to observe practice and ask what is happening. The next stage is to compare this against explicit standards based on scientific evidence on what is reasonable practice. Usually this comparison demonstrates room for improvement and the need to implement change. It is essential to close the loop of the cycle by ensuring that the information and assessment are used to good effect and not abandoned as 'orphan data'. The end product of audit is not the demonstration of problems, nor the suggestion of solutions but the implementation of appropriate change.

Applying audit to clinical specialties

National guidance

General direction on the organization and structuring of medical audit has been issued by the various departments of health for both hospital and community health services and for primary health care. For example, for England, HC(91)2[7] outlined the arrangements which health authorities and NHS trusts were required to make in order to ensure that a framework for medical audit was in place by April 1991. It defined the relevant tasks of regional health authorities and local medical audit committees and the implications for medical education and training. The equivalent guidance for general practice was issued in HC(90)15[8]. The specific methods and topics for audit were not pre-scribed nationally but were left to the discretion of the professions and many of the Royal colleges and national professional organizations took the opportunity to issue their own guidance on these matters. Guidelines have been less readily forthcoming on interdisciplinary clinical practice such as palliative care.

Organization

A number of relationships need to be clarified at national, regional and local levels. First, it is necessary to identify a local peer group and to recognize that its composition may vary according to the subject under discussion. Second, it is necessary to clarify the relationship between the clinical peer group and those who are managerially accountable for quality within a provider unit or indeed the role of the quality group in relation to purchasers and contracts. Third, it is necessary to identify the relationship between the clinical peer group and regional specialty groups which may act as a network of experience in audit to share methods and compare results and to organize relevant training. These interrelationships are not easily defined within single disciplines let alone among the variety of professions and users concerned with palliative care. However this is resolved, it is essential that each audit group defines the topic of each audit, who will be participating, how the results will be acted upon and who will have access to detailed findings and at what level of aggregation.

Methods

Audit should involve the objective peer review of patterns of care sensitive to the expectations of patients and other clinical disciplines and based on scientific evidence of good clinical practice.

- The specialty should have a prospective programme of audit defining frequency and duration of meetings, the range of methods to be used and linkage with other specialties or other units.
- Cases for review should be selected randomly or by pre-agreed criteria.
- Patterns of practice, quantified where possible, should be compared with explicit guidelines.
- Guidelines should be agreed locally but should be generally consistent with regional and national advice and with the body of scientific knowledge.
- Methods chosen for audit should be locally appropriate; they may include a combination of:
    i   random record review: individual cases reviewed by an independent clinician according to agreed parameters
    ii general review of statistics: examination of routinely provided data on key measures of workload, access, process and outcome of care
    iii specific review of adverse events: examination of individual cases identified by specified criteria such as death, complications or errors
    iv topic review: detailed quantified analysis (retrospective, concurrent or prospective) of an agreed clinically significant subject, eg by criterion-based audit or by patient satisfaction survey.

Resources

Clinical staff should be provided with the time, data, technical and clerical assistance, library support and training required to fulfil the agreed programme of audit:

- sessional time should be identified in clinical staff contracts according to the frequency, duration and location of meetings, as well as the preparation and follow-up required of individual clinicians
- the frequency, format and scope of routine statistical data provided to the specialty on resources, activity and results should be defined locally with the service managers
- minimum reference data for audit purposes include accurate, timely and complete listings of diagnoses (primary and secondary), procedures and complications

- clinical staff should ensure that diagnoses, complications and procedures are recorded accurately and promptly for clinical data capture
- technical and clerical assistance should be available for retrieving and abstracting records and for collecting, tabulating and presenting data required for the agreed programme of audit
- the clinical library service should ensure rapid access to published literature on audit methods and on effective medical care, to unpublished literature on organization and methods of audit, and to regional and national specialty libraries and resource centres
- training in audit methods should be available to all clinical staff and audit assistants.

The future prospects

Several growing pressures are likely to influence the future development of audit. These come from other specialties, managers, purchasers and particularly from patients.

The first challenge of developing medical audit into multidisciplinary clinical audit is less of an issue in palliative care than it is in more medically dominated specialties, although it still requires a reconciliation of differing views on care planning and the scientific basis of clinical practice.

Second, there is an increasing tendency for managers, many of whom see no tangible signs of benefits emerging from clinical audit, to want to direct the audit agenda and to see the detailed results; this underlines a need for prior agreement on confidentiality of audit data and on explicit specifications of the purpose, nature and products of clinical audit in return for the resources invested.

Third, there is a growing concern among the population as a whole to know not only that there is a general mechanism for ensuring clinical quality but also to know specific results and performance measures for individual units; the most constructive professional response to this pressure may well be to empower patients by providing them with clear indications of the level of service which they could reasonably expect and by which they may judge for themselves the quality of clinical practice.

However, it must be recognized that there will remain areas of technical competence in which both patients and managers will have to rely upon the professions to regulate themselves – and to demonstrate that they are doing so. The clinical professions still have the opportunity to take this initiative and to work constructively with patients and managers in improving quality. This requires co-operation locally and networking and leadership nationally.

References

1 Joint Working Party on the Organisation of Medical Work in Hospitals (1974) *Third Report (Cogwheels Report)*. London: HMSO.

2 Report of the Committee on Nursing (1972) *Briggs Report*. London: HMSO.

3 Committee of Enquiry into Competence to Practise (Chairman: E A J Alment) (1976) *Competence to Practise*. London: HMSO.

4 *Royal Commission on the National Health Service* (1979) London: HMSO.

5 Griffiths R (1983) *Department of Health and Social Security NHS Management Inquiry*. London: DHSS.

6 The Secretaries of State for Health (1989) *Working for Patients* (White Paper). London: HMSO.

7 *Medical Audit in Hospital and Community Health Services* (1990) HC(91)2. London: DoH.

8 Department of Health (1990) *Medical Audit in Family Practitioner Services*, HC(90)15. London: DoH.

2

Clinical Audit for Palliative Care

IRENE HIGGINSON

Introduction

This chapter gives a definition of palliative care, and discusses how and where audit of palliative care can occur. Options for audit, some benefits and disadvantages, differences between audit of palliative care in hospitals, hospices and the community, and between professional groups are highlighted.

Palliative care: what does it mean?

The word palliative is derived from the Latin word 'pallium' meaning a cloak or cover. In its most literal use, it refers to the provision of active care for a person whose condition is not responsive to curative treatment[1]. Over the last 20 years the provision of quality care to patients with advanced progressive disease has been a growing concern for health, voluntary and social services. Many countries have developed or expanded palliative services[2], often closely bound to the hospice movement.

A modern definition of palliative care is:

'active total care offered to a patient with a progressive disease and their family when it recognised that the illness is no longer curable, in order to concentrate on the quality of life and the alleviation of distressing symptoms within the framework of a co-ordinated service. Palliative care neither hastens nor postpones death, it provides relief from pain and other distressing symptoms, integrates the psychological and spiritual aspects of care. In addition it offers a support system to help relatives and friends cope during the patient's illness and in bereavement'[1]

'Family' is used as a general term to cover closely attached individuals, whatever their legal status.

In many countries patients spend most of their last year of life at home but, as well as the primary care team, patients and families are likely to have care from hospitals. Hospices, specialist palliative care teams, Macmillan nurses, Marie Curie nurses, nursing homes, residential homes and social services can often also contribute to care. Therefore, palliative care affects many professionals who may wish to audit their work.

Different professionals and audit

Holistic multiprofessional care underpins the philosophy of many palliative care programmes. Such an approach is implied by the term 'within the framework of a co-ordinated service' from the definition of palliative care given above. However, initially in health care, separate medical and nursing audits developed (see Box 2.1). An alternative

---

Box 2.1: Definitions of various types of audit

Medical audit
The systematic critical analysis of the quality of medical care including the procedures used for diagnosis and treatment, the use of resources and the resulting outcome and quality of life for the patient (see Chapter 1).

Clinical audit
The systematic critical analysis of the quality of clinical care including the procedures used for diagnosis and treatment, the use of resources and the resulting outcome and quality of life for the patient.

Clinical audit is like medical audit but involves all professionals and volunteers, rather than only doctors.

Nursing audit
The methods by which nurses compare their actual practice against pre-agreed guidelines and identify areas for improving their care. Examples of nursing audit include Monitor[3], Phaneuf's[4] and Qualpac[5].

Prospective audit
The standards and measures are agreed at the start and are recorded on patients and families during their care.

Retrospective audit
Looks back at the care of patients using either the clinical notes and extracting the information or by asking families.

Box 2.2: Single professional versus clinical audit

Separate goals

Nursing audit
Medical audit
Social work audit
Volunteer audit
Physiotherapy audit

Common goals

Team audit
Clinical audit

approach is to adopt clinical audit, which includes all relevant professionals, although this is possible only if the goals of care are common to those involved in the audit. Where goals differ it may be more appropriate to undertake audit of different professionals (*see* Box 2.2) and then regularly bring together the results of any medical, nursing or other audits.

Whether carried out by single professional groups or by a multi-professional team, audit is a cycle where standards or goals are set, compared with reality by observing practice, then results are fed back to improve practice and set new standards and repeat the audit cycle (*see* Figure 2.1). Clinical audit can begin at any point in the cycle – the cycle varies – but most people choose to begin by either setting standards or by reviewing practice.

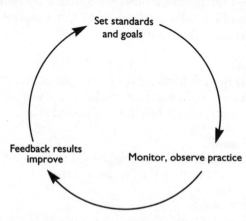

Figure 2.1: The audit cycle

Different settings

Audit carried out in the community, hospitals or hospices may need to be slightly different because of different goals of care and the numbers and types of patients and families receiving care. Each year an average general practitioner (GP) will care for 10 to 20 patients who will die that year, some of them dying suddenly. Many of the methods and measures described later can be adapted for different settings but it may be that only a small part of the measure should be used. For example, the approach taken in Chapter 10 of using the views of bereaved family members has been used by GPs[6]. Equally, a few items of the Support Team Assessment Schedule (*see* page 35), the Edmonton Symptom Assessment Scale (*see* page 61), and Palliative Care Core Standards (*see* Chapter 9) could be used by hospital or community staff.

Why audit palliative care?

Improving the quality of their palliative care is a goal of most professionals. There are also external pressures to improve the quality of health care. Individuals in today's society are much more conscious of their rights to demand high quality care and, through government, wish to ensure that professionals are accountable for the health care they provide.

Antipathy to audit is based on various arguments such as:

● there is no problem since palliative care is of a high quality and is self-auditing
● palliative care cannot be measured
● resources, information and time are not available
● audit looks back at practice which has gone, not the problems which lie ahead (*see* Figure 2.2).

However, there is good evidence that palliative practice varies from one part of the country to another, even in simple aspects such as staffing levels, the catchment populations, the operational policies and the throughput[7]. We need to know for which patients palliative care is most effective and which models of care work best. Those providing and those purchasing palliative services will need to know which interventions and in what combination, for what kinds of patients and families, work best in their locality (*see* Chapter 4). Examples of problems in health care which can or are being addressed by audit are shown in Box 2.3.

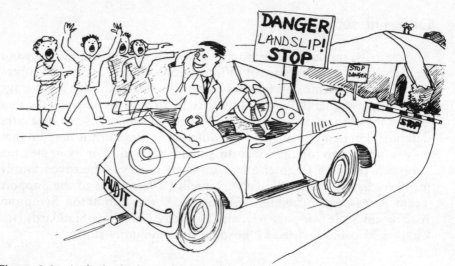

Figure 2.2: Audit looks back, by David Perman

Box 2.3: Examples of problems in health care which can or are being addressed by audit

Communication: a quarter of all cases of malpractice handled by medical defence organizations involved a failure of communication between professionals or between them and their patients.

Drug interactions: 24% of elderly people admitted to a teaching hospital were on drugs which were contraindicated or interacting.

The Confidential Enquiry into Perioperative Deaths, a major audit of all deaths within 30 days of surgical operation in three regions, indicated that some deaths could have been prevented, by delaying operation until the morning with a more experienced surgeon or by stabilizing the medical problems before surgery.

Source: Shaw, 1992[8]

Benefits of palliative care audit

Palliative care audit can benefit patients and families in the following ways:

- identifying problems in practice and, through the audit cycle, improving care will mean that future patients and families should not suffer the same problems

- aiming staff time and resources on aspects of care which work, rather than those which do not, means that patients and their families receive the most up-to-date and effective care
- prospective audits directly benefit patients and families in care during the audit. The systematic assessment of patients and families in care will mean that:
  - i   aspects of care are less likely to be overlooked
  - ii   there is a more holistic approach to care
  - iii   new staff have a clearer understanding of what they should assess
- audit helps most patients and families receiving palliative care because it looks at routine practice rather than at a few 'special' cases. Quite apart from mistakes, suboptimal care may be due to professional or administrative problems which tend to escape anecdotal case reviews.

Audit can help any services providing palliative care in the following ways:

- staff are able to monitor and review the quality of their work and seek ways of improving it
- audit provides a systematic way of thinking about objectives and outcomes of care
- audit identifies areas where care is effective and where it is not
- the problems of patients and families are considered in more detail.

Audit is important for education and training because the structured review allows analysis, comparision and evaluation of individual performance; it promotes adherence to local clinical policies and offers opportunity for publication of results. Educational programmes can be constructed to meet the demonstrated needs of individuals or groups.

Audit may also be required for the recognition of training posts: Royal colleges and faculties increasingly seek evidence of formally organized review and could withdraw recognition from departments that do not provide this.

Dangers of not auditing care

Hospices and palliative services bring new therapies, such as new treatments for symptoms, support and counselling services or complementary therapies. However, new therapies and approaches must be evaluated and audited to determine if and with whom these are useful otherwise resources and the patient's time will be wasted. There is a great danger of concentrating only on current concerns without reviewing previous failings and using the findings to plan improved care

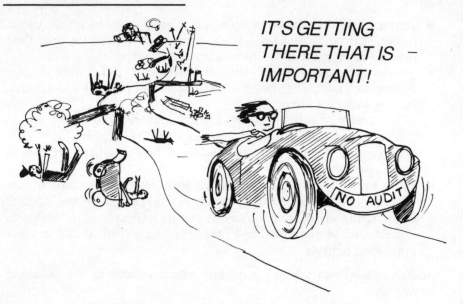

Figure 2.3: No audit, by David Perman

in the future. Failure to look back at the road behind can be dangerous (*see* Figure 2.3). The costs of not auditing are as important as the benefits of auditing. These include:

- extra inappropriate treatment, which wastes the patients' and families' time and resources on such treatment, as well as wasting staff time and resources. Such resources could be used where they may be more effective
- uncontrolled symptoms may cause admission to a hospice or hospital, or delay discharge. Most significantly this causes suffering to the patient, family and staff
- there may be extra inappropriate services, for example unnecessary outpatient attendances.

Conclusions

Palliative care – the total active care for a patient with progressive incurable disease and their family – involves many professionals. Audit can benefit patients, families and professionals by identifying failings and improving the quality of care. However, as described in the previous chapter, taking part in audit has a cost in terms of staff time and resources and therefore it needs to be carried out as effectively as possible. The remainder of this book provides examples of clinical audit in palliative care which could be adapted by those professionals beginning audit, and it provides information for those who wish to compare their approach and results with others.

References

1 Standing Medical Advisory Committee and Standing Nursing and Midwifery Advisory Committee (1992) *The principles and provision of palliative care*. Joint report of the Standing Medical Advisory Committee and Standing Nursing and Midwifery Advisory Committee, London.

2 Higginson I (1993) Palliative care: a review of past changes and future trends. *Journal of Public Health Medicine* 15(1): 3–8.

3 Goldstone LA, Ball JA and Collier MM (1983) *Monitor – an index of the quality of nursing services on acute medical and surgical wards.* Newcastle-Upon-Tyne Polytechnic Products Ltd.

4 Phaneuf M (1976) *The nursing audit.* New York: Appleton-Century-Crofts.

5 Wandelt MA and Ager J (1974) *Quality patient care scale (Qualpac).* New York: Appleton-Century-Crofts.

6 Berlin A, Spencer JA, Bhopal RS and van Zwanenberg D (1992) Audit of the deaths in general practice: a pilot study of the critical incident technique. *Quality in Health Care* 1: 231–235.

7 Kirkham S (1992) Bed occupancy, patient throughput and size of independent hospice units in the UK. *Palliative Medicine* 6: 47–53.

8 Shaw CD (1992) *Speciality medical audit.* London: King's Fund Centre.

3

Clinical Audit: Getting Started, Keeping Going

IRENE HIGGINSON

Introduction

Audit can be distinguished from simple review of patients because it should be regular, include cases selected at random, rather than selected because they are unusual and have systematic criteria for success[1]. This requires more work than the occasional review of an interesting case. It is also potentially more threatening because the aims of audit are to identify areas where care is not meeting agreed standards, to change practice to improve care and then to repeat the audit cycle. To succeed audit itself must be effective and staff need to feel a tangible benefit which is worth the time and effort devoted to audit. A way of assessing staff's views about the usefulness of audit is described in Chapter 15. Some of the common guidance for successful audit[1,2], and experiences in failures and success, are drawn together in this chapter.

Starting audit

Starting audit can be a very difficult process. However, the initial stages of audit are very important and often determine whether the audit is successful later. The mnemonic 'SPREE' brings together some guidance.

- Small. Audit should be cheap and simple and cause a minimum disruption to care. It is better to begin small and then grow when audit is more established.
- Plan. There needs to be a clear plan of the audit and commitment to it from all staff. This will require leadership from senior staff, but also participation of all staff, and a clear view of how the audit will

evolve, its method, and when it will be reviewed. Ideally there needs to be some discussion from all staff at an early stage, *see* Chapters 5, 7, 14, 15 and 16 for further ideas.

- **Regular.** Audit meetings, the collection of information and the review of results must occur regularly otherwise these become lost in other aspects of care.
- **Exchange.** It helps to exchange ideas within the audit group and where possible with other audit groups learning each other's mistakes and successes.
- **Enjoy.** Perhaps the most important aspect. The intention of audit must be – and be seen to be – educational and relevant to clinical care. It is important that staff do not see audit as a threat, they should feel ownership of the audit. This is helped if participation is voluntary and if the staff feel they have had a hand in developing or choosing the methods.

What to measure?

Chapter 1 outlined some of the methods of audit. Audit also needs a successful way of measuring the aspect to be considered. Some key features are included in the mnemonic 'BRAVE'.

- **Borrow** standards, methods and measures from others to save time and resources if at all possible, then adapt these to local circumstances. As later chapters will demonstrate the development of standards and measures can often be very time consuming, taking up to a year and sometimes longer. If standards or measures already exist it is often expedient to use these or adapt them to local needs.
- **Reliable** measures or criteria are needed if more than one person will assess the standards, otherwise time will be wasted and the results can mean little. Reliability refers to the stability and consistency of information provided by the measure, also sometimes referred to as the precision of the measurement[3]. It is reflected by the repeatability of measures. A measure is reliable to the extent that repeated measures under constant conditions will give the same result. Reliability can be tested by the test-retest method, which compares the ratings of different assessors or the same assessor over a period of time. Other ways of assessing reliability include developing two measures simultaneously and comparing their assessments of the same subjects, or testing for the internal consistency (or homogeneity) of a scale[4]. Internal consistency is important, if a measure contains a series of items, each of which is supposed to reflect one underlying construct such as quality of life. One test of internal consistency is split-half reliability. Here items are subdivided into

two sub-scales and the scores are correlated with each other. However, there may be many different ways that the items can be subdivided (odd numbers versus even numbers, first half versus second half, etc), and the reliability co-efficient may vary greatly depending on how the items are divided. A better test is Chronbach's alpha[5], which gives the average of all possible split-half reliabilities of the scale, although a computer is normally needed for this calculation. In both tests, the number of items in the scale must be accounted for in the final calculation.

Reliability can be enhanced by using the measure in controlled conditions, by ensuring that assessors are adequately trained, by using unambiguous items, and by providing unambiguous rating instructions[6].

- Appropriate standards and measures are needed, so that staff feel these are truly assessing the work in their setting.
- Valid measures and criteria which accurately measure what the investigator sets out to measure are important if audit is to be effective and to achieve the main goal of audit – improving the care for the patient and family. Validity has various components, see Box 3.1. If a measure is shown to be valid, it must have at least some degree of reliability; however, a measure may be totally reliable but not valid at all!
- Easy. The methods must be simple enough to be understood and to apply in routine practice. Ideally information for audit should be collected in monthly, weekly or daily practice. Boyle and Torrance[7] proposed that, to maximize its usefulness, a measure should:
  - i   be simple to apply
  - ii   be acceptable to its respondents
  - iii be brief and inexpensive to administer
  - iv   use pre-coded response categories
  - v   use an explicit time period of assessment (eg today, the last week or month)
  - vi   use clear unambiguous instructions for respondents
  - vii *not* require prior access to or use of clinical or laboratory services.

Whose assessment?

Whether the patient, professional, family members or external professionals makes the assessments is often determined by the aspect of care being audited. Advantages and limitations of each approach are outlined below, and are discussed further in Chapter 10.

Box 3.1: Definitions of basic terms in validity. Compiled from definitions given by Streiner and Norman (1989)[4], Bowling (1988)[8], Abramson (1990)[9], Moser and Kalton (1971)[6], Cronbach (1990)[5].

Term	Definition
Validity	The success of a scale in measuring what it sets out to measure.
Face validity	Whether the scale appears relevant, reasonable and is acceptable to those using the test.
Content validity	The items should contain the common thread of what is under study and sample all the relevant or important content or domains in a balanced way.
Consensus validity	When a number of experts agree measurement is valid.
Criterion validity	Whether there is a correlation between the measure under consideration and another measure or event which is suitable for use as a criterion of validity (a gold standard).
	The best criterion is one which has higher face validity than the measure being tested and/or which has been tested previously and found to be of high criterion validity[9].
	Criterion validity can be tested concurrently (concurrent validity) or by the accurate prediction of future events (predictive validity).
Construct validity	On the basis of theoretical considerations the researcher postulates the types and degrees of associations between the scale and other variables, and then examines these associations to determine if they confirm the expectations[6].
	Construct validity is needed when gold standard measures are not available to test for criterion validity. This is common when attempting to measure something which is not readily observed, such as anxiety or some symptoms[4].

Patients

- Taking assessments directly from the person who is dying would seem to give the most valid information.
- It may be an intrusion but in one study the relatives reported that they believed dying patients were willing to help in research, often in the hope that this would help others[10]. Fallowfield *et al.* found that most breast cancer patients reported that taking part in a psychological study was a helpful extension to their treatment[11].
- The reliability and completeness of assessments from severely ill patients have been questioned. Ward[12] and Lunt and Neale[13] found that, of patients in hospice and home care settings, only one half to one third of patients in care survived and were well enough to be interviewed. Maguire[14] warned that a far greater proportion of cancer patients than usually realized may have impaired attention, concentration or memory, which can seriously affect recordings[15]. If the most ill patients cannot be assessed by interview this is a potential source of bias.

Relatives or friends

- Relatives are not as difficult to interview as severely ill patients.
- Assessments are limited to cases where a close relative or friend exists.
- Assessments may be affected by their own process of grief[16]. Epstein *et al.* tested for correlations between the ratings of 60 subjects and found that correlations between patients and their carers were good if they were in close contact, but if the subjects were in poor health, or there was little contact, or the subjects and carers lived apart, significant correlations were not found[17]. A study comparing the assessments of relatives in the bereavement period showed that these did not correlate with the assessments of patients made during their life[18]. Cartwright and Seale compared patient and bereaved relatives' or close friends' assessments of symptoms and services[19]. Mean squared congruence ranged from 0.00 (bad temper) to 0.67 (constipation). Relatives tended to be more critical of services and to report more symptoms. Parkes suggested that relatives may over-report symptoms when patients are at home[16].

External assessors

- These can provide an independent view of the patient's circumstances, free from many of the biases of professionals or the family.
- They may cause intrusion and may interfere with clinical practice.
- They may be too costly for audit.

Professionals

- Assessors may be biased by their own expectations and hopes. Slevin[20], Hinton[21] and Wilkes[22] have found that hospital and community staff gave different assessments of quality of life compared with dying patients themselves.
- They have the advantage of being able to provide data on all of the patients in their care.

There is no ideal choice of assessor. However, it is important not to change from one assessor to another (eg from patient to carer), unless you know how well the assessors agree or correlate.

A long way to gold standard measures

Auditors should not become over-confident in their measures. It is much easier to set out standards than to embody these in appropriate, acceptable and effective forms of audit, especially as we move from things that can be counted to the hard-to-measure qualitative aspects of care[23]. Mount and Scott likened measuring palliative care to measuring the beauty of a rose[24]. They commented:

'Consider the rose. You can weigh it, photograph it, categorise it, measure its height, petal size and number of thorns, not to mention the ratio of thorns to height. The mean and standard deviation of the measures can then be determined. . . . The colour may be determined by spectroscopic analysis; the chemical composition defined, the light refraction from the dewdrop on the petal measured and aroma quantified (perhaps a group of descriptors similar to the Melzack Pain Ratings Index could be devised). . . .
. . . . Although we would like to measure the beauty of a rose or to quantify the sense of fulfilment of a dying person, we do not yet have the tools.'

We have more tools in 1993 than in 1983 but there is still much work to be done, developing, testing and validating appropriate measures for the less tangible aspects of care, and where quality for one patient may be loathsome for another (*see* Figure 3.1).

Feedback, review and repeating the audit cycle

This can be a difficult time when many audits can break down and be abandoned. A clear plan in the early stages helps to prevent this, the following guidance in the mnemonic 'ARISE' may also assist.

- Analyse often so that the results are considered early, not when a large amount of data has been collected.

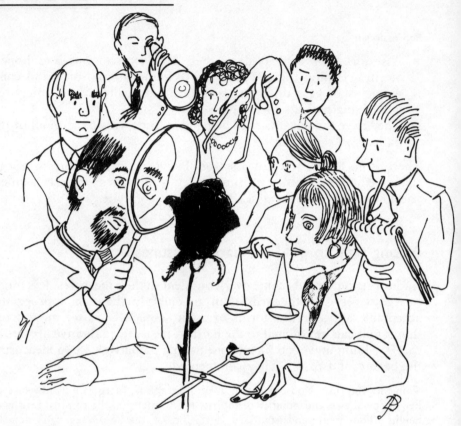

Figure 3.1: Consider a rose, by David Perman

- Review the audit results, the progress of the audit, and the positive and negative effects of the audit on staff and patients to plan the future developments.
- Instigate change both in working practice and in the audit method used, even if the changes are relatively small, before the audit cycle is repeated.
- Set new standards – to be monitored in a new audit cycle.
- Effect new cycle, building on the results of the previous audit.

Conclusions

Developing a clear plan of audit and maintaining enthusiasm is an important, but often overlooked, step. Measures used in audit need to be sensitive, valid and reliable if the audit results are to be of any value. Acting on feedback from results is where many audits fall down. Small audits with frequent feedback may be more successful, and ways of achieving these are discussed in the later chapters of this book.

References

1 Shaw C (1989) *Medical audit. A hospital handbook*. London: King's Fund Centre.

2 Shaw C (1992) *Speciality medical audit*. London: King's Fund Centre.

3 Nunnally JC (1978) *Psychometric theory*. New York: McGraw Hill (2nd edition).

4 Streiner DL and Norman GR (1989) *Health measurement scales. A practical guide to their development and use*. Oxford: Oxford University Press.

5 Cronbach LJ (1990) *Essentials of psychological testing*. New York: Harper and Row (5th edition).

6 Moser CA and Kalton G (1971) *Survey methods in social investigation*. London: Heinemann (2nd edition).

7 Boyle MH and Torrance GW (1984) Developing multiattribute health indexes. *Medical Care* **22**(11): 1045–57.

8 Bowling A (1991) *Measuring health. A review of quality of life measurement scales*. Milton Keynes: Open University.

9 Abramson JH (1990) Survey methods in community medicine. *Epidemiological studies, programme evaluation, clinical trials*. Edinburgh: Churchill Livingstone (4th edition).

10 Mor V, Greer DS and Kastenbaum R (1988) *The hospice experiment*. Baltimore: Johns Hopkins University Press.

11 Fallowfield LJ, Baum M and Maguire GP (1987) Do psychological studies upset patients? *Journal of the Royal Society of Medicine* **80**: 59.

12 Ward AWM (1985) *Home care services for the terminally ill*. Sheffield: Medical Care Research Unit, Department of Community Medicine, University of Sheffield Medical School.

13 Lunt B and Neale C (1985) *A comparision of hospice and hospital care for terminally ill cancer patients and their families. A comparision of care goals set by staff (Paper D)*. Southampton: Department of Community Medicine, University of Southampton.

14 Maguire P (1980) Monitoring the quality of life in cancer patients and their relatives. In Symington T, Williams AE and McVie JG (eds.). *Cancer: assessment and monitoring*. London: Churchill Livingstone, 40–52.

15 Miller E (1992) Basic principles of neuropsychological assessment. In Crawford J, McKinlay W and Parker D (eds.). *Practice and principles of neuropsychological assessment*. Hove, Sussex: Laurence Erlbaum.

16 Parkes CM (1985) Terminal care: home, hospital, or hospice? *Lancet* i: 155–7.

17 Epstein AM, Hall JA, Tognetti J, Son LH and Conant L (1989) Using proxies to evaluate quality of life. Can they provide valid information about patient's health status and satisfaction with medical care. *Medical Care* 27(3): S91–S98.

18 Ahmedzai S, Morton A, Reid JT and Stevenson RD (1988) Quality of death from lung cancer: patients' reports and relatives' retrospective opinions. *In*: Watson M, Greer S and Thomas C (eds.). *Psychosocial Oncology*. Oxford: Pergamon Press.

19 Cartwright A and Seale C (1990) *The natural history of a survey: an account of the methodological issues encountered in a study of life before death*. London: King Edward's Hospital Fund.

20 Slevin ML, Plant H, Lynch D, Drinkwater J and Gregory WM (1988) Who should measure quality of life – the doctor or the patient? *British Journal of Cancer* 57: 109–12.

21 Hinton J (1979) A comparison of places and policies for terminal care. *Lancet* i: 29–32.

22 Wilkes E (1984) Dying now: *Lancet* i: 950–2.

23 Ford G (1990) Constructive audit. *Palliative Medicine* 4(1): Editorial.

24 Mount BM and Scott JF (1983) Whither hospice evaluation? *Journal of Chronic Diseases* 36: 731–6.

4

Clinical Audit – Everyone's Business?

JANET DOYLE

Introduction

There is a convergence of interest amongst NHS policymakers, purchasing authorities and statutory and voluntary providers of palliative care in sustaining recognized good practice and identifying areas for improvement. Clinical audit is expected to support each of these groups in their respective decisions by establishing standards of clinical care and systematically measuring performance. This chapter considers the purchasers' view of the process and outcome of clinical audit, and thus might offer providers of palliative care services insights into the priorities and main concerns of those who commission their services. The interest of the current regional health authorities in clinical audit is also considered as part of the context within which palliative care services are delivered.

The audit of change

Clinical audit takes place against a background of rapid change in all areas of the health service, including the culture of the market, development of trusts, GP fund-holding, The Patients' Charter, the *Health of the Nation*, community care and the focus on public and consumer involvement. It would be understandable for health care professionals to feel overwhelmed by the pace and scope of such change but, in providing for the establishment of standards and systematic measurement, clinical audit can help providers and purchasers during a period of change. In addition, since the principles of palliative care are also the key to good health care in general, understanding developed through the audit of palliative care may make a significant contribution to improvements in care provided to patients, their families and friends in other sectors of the health service.

Rising priority

Until recently, the terms palliative care and terminal care have been equated with care of those with advanced cancer, but today there is wider recognition of the need to achieve greater equality of care for those suffering from other life-threatening diseases. Care is to be based on need not disease, and it has been suggested there should be 'palliative care for all'.

In *Health of the Nation – First Steps for the NHS*, under 'Cancer' (one of the five target areas) palliative care and its audit are considered to be one of a range of possible activities for the NHS to start the process of implementing the *Health of the Nation* strategy[1]. District health authorities (DHAs) are required to ensure that data are available to measure the level and quality of service provision, and it is envisaged that this will precede the commissioning of palliative care based on principles developed nationally[2]. Such care may include, for example:

- general care and support services for the patients and family
- symptom control (eg pain, cough, breathlessness)
- specialist palliative treatment (eg radiotherapy, chemotherapy and surgery)
- bereavement care and counselling[3].

National recommendations

Preceding *First Steps for the NHS*, a Joint Report of the Standing Medical Advisory Committee (SMAC) and Standing Nursing and Midwifery Advisory Committee (SNMAC)[4], made a series of recommendations to the Secretary of State in the light of rapid and often patchy developments in the provision of palliative care services. It was recognized that health authority support for palliative care services had invariably been unco-ordinated and unplanned, and that an authoritative consensus on the appropriate level and quality of services provided, and how they may be purchased or monitored, was missing. The remit for this work was to consider the whole range of palliative care services, whether in the voluntary or statutory sector, within the context of the whole spectrum of need, regardless of the cause of the anticipated death.

The main proposals of the SMAC and SNMAC report embrace issues of education and strategic planning as a foundation for the development of the highest standards of palliative and terminal care in all settings. Recognized principles and examples of good practice, ostensibly stimulated within the voluntary movement, should be incorporated at all levels of the NHS. Audit and operational research are crucial to this objective and, whilst it is recognized that examples of good practice, audit and research exist, until now work has not been either widely published or available nationally. Standards of care and outcome measures that are understood should become a regular part of practice rather than being perceived, as sometimes is the case, to be an optional extra. The intention is for palliative care services to be integrated more with the function of primary health care teams with specialists providing advice and acting as a resource.

One of the general objectives within the report is that palliative care should be received as a continuous part of health care and not as a distinct or separate service, and that what is learnt through the evaluation of care in one setting should be transferred to other settings. Purchasers will be looking for evidence that attempts are being made to do so.

The future

Achieving the aims set out in the SMAC and SNMAC report within available resources will be a gradual process, and the report's recommendations can be used to influence current approaches and future palliative care strategies. It is important that the developmental nature of clinical audit is recognized, so that change is encouraged where appropriate, as well as the maintenance of good, effective practice.

Regions' view

The regional health authorities' role in clinical audit involves establishing the criteria for distribution and monitoring of centrally funded grants for medical and clinical audit and, in addition, until the year 1994–5, allocating specific funds to voluntary hospices and specialist palliative care services, towards their running costs[5].

Increasingly, emphasis is on establishing clinical audit strategies that fully reflect multi-professional interests and integrate the consumer and public perspective. In a number of regions, previously separate committees for medical audit and nursing and therapy audit have been amalgamated and joint bids for multi-professional projects are thus encouraged.

In monitoring outcomes of audit activity, there is often a lack of evidence to demonstrate that the findings have resulted in any change in practice or, where change has been instigated, that re-auditing is planned. The audit loop or cycle is not completed. To do so effectively, the management and psychology of change should be addressed and resourced within strategic plans. If not, it would be too easy for audit to be viewed merely as a paper exercise, or another new fad.

Regions' activity can provide support for the process of change by assisting productive networking of providers with similar interests, the identification and sharing of good practice, and the provision by professionals specializing in audit of advice and guidance to providers.

Philosophy supporting clinical audit

Organizational commitment to clinical audit can be expressed through a corporate contractual objective such as that between regions and purchasing authorities. It is anticipated that purchasers will include a requirement for clinical audit when commissioning palliative care services and will address the infrastructure and staff time required to support it, as well as integrating a public perspective. In addition there will be specific standards for quality, stipulated in contractual agreements, which are relevant to palliative care situations. These may include issues such as privacy and dignity, the provision of information, tissue damage, nutrition and dietary requirements.

Different and contrasting views are often held by health care workers about what the term audit means and regions and purchasers would therefore look for evidence of activity that supports the development of a common understanding between different professional groups. The hallmark of palliative care is teamwork, with professionals sharing assessment and decision-making in order to support an holistic approach[6]. Multi-professional audit, together with commitment to review collectively uni-professional audit results, will support this philosophy.

Research is often confused with audit by medical and clinical staff. Whereas the findings of research, for example, which contrasts two forms of treatment may be used to establish standards for audit, it does not itself constitute audit.

Purchasing authorities are increasingly including an appropriate understanding by all clinical staff within their quality standards, as in for example North West Anglia Health Authority's document *Standards and quality for contracts*:

'The principles of clinical audit should be understood by all clinical staff, and there should be evidence from Provider Units to show that appropriate training programmes have been established to prepare staff, with a view to implementing clinical audit within an agreed strategy. There should be evidence of speciality specific standards with appropriate outcome measures.' (*Reprinted by kind permission of North West Anglia Health Authority.*)

This extract also highlights an expectation that specific standards and outcomes for palliative care will be developed.

Purchaser's priorities

District health authorities' principle function is to secure high quality health care for the resident population, based on assessment of need and provided within available resources. Knowledge and information discovered through audit provide objective evidence that a service is working towards the most effective use of clinical resources and aims to improve the quality of care. This will obviously be significant when different services are competing for contracts.

In setting contracts with palliative care services and hospices, purchasers are likely to incorporate a requirement for audit. This may include a number of areas such as unit policies, staff training, staff sickness and turnover, referral and access patterns, quality visits, contract monitoring, registration and inspection[6]. In future, audit will be costed for in-contract agreements and quality assurance monitoring will embrace evidence of audit. Standards for quality and audit will be required in contract specifications and subsequently will need to be included and costed in the service providers' business plan.

In addition to clinical audit, purchasers will be concerned with the audit of organizational structures, which can act as a potential proxy for actual clinical outcomes. There are enormous limitations with this approach as actual outcomes are not evaluated, but it does take account of the volume of monitoring for which the purchasers are responsible, as well as the dearth of definable standards and lack of knowledge disseminated of those standards that do exist in palliative care.

A quality framework originally produced by a group of regional nurses funded by Cancer Relief Macmillan Fund[7] has been adapted and adopted by a number of regional and purchasing authorities, and considers the following standards:

- values and objectives
- policy
- research and development
- level of service provision
- education and training
- direct patient and family care
- health promotion

- multidisciplinary teams
- continuity of care
- quality assurance.

This framework can address the variation, which may exist in the organizational capacity of units to sustain clinical care, by identifying desirable resources and activities that should be the foundation of that care[8]. Progress towards meeting these standards can be assessed and targets for action can be identified. This tool has been developed for use in any setting, generic or specialist. An organizational audit designed specifically for specialist palliative care services by a working party funded by Cancer Relief Macmillan Fund is currently being piloted[9].

There is increasing interest amongst purchasers in identifying outcome measures that demonstrate health gain, the focus of purchasing activity. In palliative care this relates to quality of life for the patient and carers rather than longevity, the indicator usually used. Collaborative work between purchasers and provider units is to be encouraged, in order to identify desirable outcomes and develop appropriate outcome measures. Such outcomes can be developed to reflect the health care trajectory of an individual, such as for the period surrounding the diagnosis of a life-threatening disease, the phase of active treatment, which may include palliation, and the terminal phase, likely to mark the final illness.

Generally, at present, information and data on outcomes of palliative care is limited and unsophisticated. One of the aims of clinical audit is to contribute to the knowledge base. Initially services may wish to scrutinize one or two relevant issues such as transfer of care, effectiveness of pain relief, range of clients for admission and client choice. These will complement the stated objectives of a palliative care service and specialists can develop standards for audit that generalists may achieve.

Patients should be able to exercise, wherever practicable, choice of provision and location of services. Purchasers may be unaware of factors, which on occasion may preclude the realization of such an objective but will require the presentation of systematic data and clear evaluation during the monitoring process. Questions that will be raised by purchasers will emulate from accepted service philosophies and other public statements, which claim to provide a specific style and quality of service. The cost effectiveness of such care will have to be balanced with all other purchasing decisions and priorities.

What are purchasers interested in?

This question was posed during a regional seminar to discuss developing contracts in palliative care. Present were heads of purchasing, directors of quality, consultants in public health and the following themes emerged. There should be a focus for audit which complements the *Health of the Nation* targets, purchasing priorities of a particular health authority, and is integrated with the research and development strategy. Purchasers need to see results, which often appear to either not exist or not to be available. It is clear that nationally a great deal of time, funding and other resources are invested in these activities and they need to be supported by protocols and a timetable with regular information being provided on how the programme is being developed.

A prevalent view, until more recently, has been for medical and clinical audit to be seen purely as an internal professional issue and interest from, and involvement of, management to be interpreted as 'muscling in on medical and clinical freedom'. This contrasts with the purchaser expectation that the focus of such investment should be to benefit and contribute to the activity of the organization and to provide evidence of change.

The key to moving towards a convergence of interest amongst purchasers and providers is collaboration, which may extend to agreeing suitable subjects for audit. It is often perceived that subjects selected are not always legitimate for audit. In some instances, this has led to purchasing authorities stipulating audit programmes, when it is preferable for plans to arise out of a dialogue between purchasers and audit committees, public health officers and other provider colleagues. Priorities will clearly not always coincide, but misunderstanding and potential conflict can be minimized by this type of approach.

Providing quality care

Provider responsibility is to maintain the level and quality of care, which has been contracted for with the purchaser, whilst remaining within income and expenditure balance. To survive, the providers' service must be:

- effective
- equitable
- efficient
- accessible
- appropriate
- responsive

and must work towards these values where they are not already met.

The mechanisms that can be utilized to feed back results to the purchasers are through formal contracting meetings and quality monitoring visits and via intermediate and summative written reports of audit activity. In practice, this should occur within a collaborative relationship and the unit concerned should court purchasers and be creative in seeking opportunities to inform them about progress and the findings of audit projects. A key message is to involve purchasers.

What information is required from providers?

Purchasers are interested in establishing the interventions that are most effective and the models of care which work best for the patients and families for whose health care they are responsible. This will lead to identifying the combination of services that should be available and for which patients and families they can be targeted. Epidemiological data, service usage and other information collated by palliative care services can assist purchasers in their decision-making.

Conclusion

There are great benefits for purchasers and providers learning together, while also understanding and respecting each other's roles. Those with a remit for quality and audit in both areas, need to have close liaison and regular dialogue. Aspects of good practice and areas of concern can be jointly considered and, where possible, priorities agreed. When it can be achieved, this level of co-operation can assist recognition of account-ability for clinical audit activity, which will lead to enhanced care for those requiring palliative care, thus adding life to years.

References

1 Department of Health (1992) NHS Management Executive – *The Health of the Nation – First Steps for the NHS*. London: HMSO.

2 Doyle JH, Webb J, Webber J and Terry V (1991) One last chance to get it right. *Health Service Journal* **101**(5251): 22–3.

3 Department of Health (1993) *The Health of the Nation, key area handbook – cancers*. London: HMSO.

4 Department of Health (1992) Joint report of the Standing Medical Advisory Committee and Standing Nursing and Midwifery Advisory Committee, *The principles and provision of palliative care*.

5 NHS Management Executive (1993) *Executive letter EL(93)14*. Hospice funding.

6 National Council for Hospice and Specialist Palliative Care Services (1992) *Quality standards, organisational and clinical audit for hospices and palliative care services*. Occasional Paper 2. London: National Council for Hospice and Specialist Palliative Care Services.

7 Harris L, Hill J, Hulme P and Pooley J (1990) Framework for care. *Health Service Journal* 100(J221): 1477.

8 King's Fund Centre (1990) *Organisational audit (accreditation, UK) – standards for an acute hospital*. London: King's Fund Centre.

9 Cancer Relief Macmillan Fund (1992) *Audit for specialist palliative care services*. London: Cancer Relief Macmillan Fund.

5

Audit Methods: A Community Schedule

IRENE HIGGINSON

Introduction

This chapter describes the development of a schedule for audit of palliative care support teams. There are 360 home support teams and a further 160 hospital support services described in the *1992 Directory of Hospice Services in the United Kingdom and Republic of Ireland*[1]. The community schedule was developed to examine the outcomes and intermediate outcomes of care (*see* Chapters 1 and 2) of these services, rather than the structure or process of care. When this work began there were no suitable measures or audits available for palliative care, therefore new ones had to be developed.

To develop the audit we first defined the goals of palliative care support teams and then from these, developed ways of measuring these goals. The resulting measure – the Support Team Assessment Schedule (STAS) – was then tested for validity, reliability (*see* Chapter 6) and practicality. The measure was used to audit the care provided by five support teams working with cancer patients, and more recently has been used in various other settings.

Methods to develop the community schedule

1. Define goals

Before any service can measure its outcome, the goals of care must be clearly defined and agreed. To ensure that the goals are relevant and appropriate to the type of care provided, the goals must be taken from views of those who are working closely with patients and families, the profession, and of course, the patients and families themselves. Box 5.1 shows how this was attempted for the community audit.

Box 5.1: The goals of palliative care were defined from:

- a review of the relevant literature
- working with palliative support teams, beginning with one team and then including the views of four other teams
- observation of the teams' work
- interviews with a few of the patients and families in care
- testing and revising a list of goals and consulting widely with other professionals and services.

---

2. Change goals into measures

Once the goals were agreed the next step was to turn these into suitable measures. There are various types of measure, for example, visual analogue scales, likert scales (where raters agree or disagree with various statements), yes/no responses, or ordinal ratings scales, such as 3 point scales and 4 point scales. Examples of these different scales can be found in other chapters. The teams tested a variety of scales for their suitability, sensitivity and ease of use.

An early version of the audit measure included 14 items relevant to palliative care[2]. In this version each item was rated 0–6 according to severity. However, we realized that three items were missing, and that the 0–6 rating scale was not suitable because intermediate points in the scale were rarely used. Therefore, the rating scale was modified to a 0–4 scale. This modification was supported by the work of McKelvie who investigated the reliability and validity of a continuous, linear analogue, and various categorized (five, seven, 11) rating scales[3]. He recommended scales with five or six categories because these were most reliable, and subjects, even when using the continuous scale, operated within five or six categories.

Definitions were then agreed for each point in the scale, for every item. The definitions needed to be unambiguous and reliable. Five teams were involved in this process. It took approximately one year to reach this stage.

The Support Team Assessment Schedule (STAS)

Box 5.2 shows the 17 items included in the STAS. The items can be simply divided into the ten which deal with the patient and family, and the seven which deal with services. They can be divided further, as below:

- physical (two items – pain control, symptom control)
- emotional (two items – patient anxiety, patient insight)

- spiritual or crisis of faith (one item – spiritual)
- families or nearest carer (two items – family anxiety, family insight)
- communication (three items – communication between patient and family, communication from professionals to patient and family, communication between professionals)
- planning for dying (two items – planning, predictability)
- social and service (three items – wasted time, practical aid, financial)
- advisory role of teams (two items – professional anxiety, advising professionals).

Box 5.2: Items in the Support Team Assessment Schedule (STAS)

Ten patient and family items

Pain control
Symptom control
Patient anxiety
Family anxiety
Patient insight
Family insight
Spiritual
Planning
Predictability
Communication between patient
  and family

Seven service items

Practical aid
Financial
Wasted time
Communication from
  professionals to patient
  and family
Communication between
  professionals
Professional anxiety
Advising professionals

Box 5.3 shows the full definitions of one item – pain control. The full definitions of STAS are shown in Appendix A (*see* page 175). The Support Team Assessment Schedule is problem orientated, and the team records the severity of each item as described and perceived by the patient and/or their family.

Box 5.3: Definition and ratings of STAS item pain control

Pain control = effect of his/her pain on the patient

Rating   Definition

0 =   None.

1 =   Occasional or grumbling single pain. Patient is not bothered to be rid of symptom.

2 =   Moderate distress, occasional bad days, pain limits some activity possible within extent of disease.

3 =   Severe pain present often. Activities and concentration markedly affected by pain.

4 =   Severe and continuous overwhelming pain. Unable to think of other matters.

Value of STAS in clinical practice

Teams wished to audit care as part of routine practice. Therefore, audit was incorporated into the normal pattern of work by including the assessment forms on a back page of the patient notes. Assessments were recorded in the notes weekly, at or just after the weekly team meeting (or ward round). As new patients were referred they were included in the audit. This meant that the number of patients who were assessed increased gradually each week until all were included.

Some clinical examples

Mrs K was a 72-year-old lady who had been diagnosed with endometrial carcinoma four years earlier and had metastasis in her brain, lung and right arm. Her STAS ratings are shown in Figure 5.1. She was referred while in hospital. Her main problems were epileptic fits and breathlessness, and she and her partner (who was moderately disabled) were very anxious. She was quite aware of her prognosis. The team identified a need to provide practical aid during care, and to advise the other professionals. The STAS ratings show how some of her problems were helped, although dyspnoea proved difficult to completely alleviate and during care she developed some pain due to destruction of soft tissue by her metastasis. She remained at home until two days before she died when she was admitted to a hospice.

Figure 5.2 shows the weekly STAS scores of a 76-year-old-man, Mr T, who had cancer of the prostrate diagnosed four years ago. His wife was partially sighted and suffered from diabetes. They lived in a groundfloor council house. When Mr T was referred, his main problems were pain due to a deep vein thrombosis, a leg ulcer and bone metastasis, and frustration because he felt he was wasting a great deal of time with radiotherapy and had done for the past year.

During care, pain due to his deep vein trombosis and to the bone metastasis were resolved but pain continued to be rated as 1 – mild, due to his ulcer. Practical needs occurred on two occasions during his care when he deteriorated. Initially there was a need to improve communication between the hospital and community staff, because the GP had not been aware of the treatment given in the hospital, and several different hospital consultants were involved.

The chart shows how the team was able to improve many of Mr T's problems, and help his wife; most of his problems were alleviated in the last few weeks before he died.

DATE:								
WEEK:	0	1	2	3	4	5	6	7
Pain control	0	1	0	1	1	1	2	
Other symptom control	3	1	2	2	1	1	1	
Patient anxiety	3	2	2	2	1	0	1	
Family anxiety	3	2	2	2	2	1	1	
Patient insight	1	1	1	1	1	1	1	
Family insight	1	1	1	1	1	1	1	
Comm. between patient and family	1	0	0	0	0	0	0	
Comm. between professionals	0	0	0	0	0	0	0	
Comm. profs to patient and family	0	0	0	0	0	0	0	
TOTAL – CORE 9 ITEMS	12	8	8	9	7	5	7	
*Planning	9(2)	2	1	1	2	1	1	
*Practical	0	2	0	0	0	0	0	
*Financial	9(1)	9(1)	1	1	1	1	1	
*Wasted time	0	0	0	0	0	0	0	
*Spiritual	9	9	9	9	9	9	9	
*Professional anxiety	2	0	0	1	0	1	1	
*Advising profs	2	2	0	0	1	0	1	
TOTAL – ALL ITEMS excluding spiritual	19	15	10	12	11	8	11	
OTHER MAIN SYMPTOM:	Epileptic Fits SOB	Anxiety SOB	SOB	SOB	SOB	SOB	SOB	
KARNOFSKY	050	060	060	060	040	040	030	
DAYS IN: home	0	5	7	7	7	7	5	
hospital	7	2	0	0	0	0	0	
hospice	0	0	0	0	0	0	2	
CONTACT WITH TEAMS: Face to face with: patient/family	1	2	1	0	1	1	2	
professionals	1	0	0	1	0	1	1	
Calls: patient/family	1	1	1	2	1	1	1	
professionals	1	2	1	2	1	1	1	
KEY TEAM WORKER:	03	05	03	2/3	02	02	03	
COMMENTS:							Died in hospice	

Figure 5.1: STAS chart for Mrs K (9 indicates a missed score)

DATE:										
WEEK:	0	1	2	3	4	5	6	7	8	9
Pain control	3	2	2	2	1	1	1	1	0	1
Other symptom control	2	1	1	1	3	1	1	2	0	0
Patient anxiety	3	2	2	1	1	1	0	0	0	0
Family anxiety	3	3	3	1	1	1	1	3	0	0
Patient insight	1	1	1	1	1	1	1	1	1	1
Family insight	1	1	1	1	1	1	1	1	0	0
Comm. between patient and family	0	0	0	0	0	0	0	0	0	0
Comm. between professionals	4	1	1	2	0	0	0	1	0	0
Comm. profs to patient and family	2	1	1	1	0	0	0	0	0	0
TOTAL – CORE 9 ITEMS	19	12	12	10	8	6	5	9	1	2
*Planning	0	0	0	0	0	0	1	2	0	0
*Practical	0	0	2	0	2	0	0	0	0	0
*Financial	0	0	0	0	0	0	0	0	0	0
*Wasted time	4	0	0	0	0	0	0	0	0	0
*Spiritual	0	0	0	0	0	0	0	0	0	0
*Professional anxiety	1	1	1	1	0	0	0	1	0	0
*Advising profs	1	4	2	1	2	1	0	1	0	1
TOTAL – ALL ITEMS	25	17	17	12	12	7	6	13	1	3
OTHER MAIN SYMPTOM:	DVT Leg ulcer	"	"	→ mobility	Urine obstruction	"	Double vision	Vomit	/	/
KARNOFSKY	060	060	060	040	040	040	040	030	020	020
DAYS IN: home	7	7	7	7	7	7	7	0	0	0
hospital	0	0	0	0	0	0	0	7	7	7
hospice	0	0	0	0	0	0	0	0	0	0
CONTACT WITH TEAMS: Face to face with: patient/family	2	2	1	1	2	2	1	2	2	3
professionals	1	1	2	0	2	0	1	1	1	0
Calls: patient/family	0	1	1	1	0	1	1	0	1	0
professionals	0	0	0	1	1	0	0	1	0	1
KEY TEAM WORKER:	02	02	02	03	02	02	05	05	02	03
COMMENTS:				→ Catheter needed	Catheter- ised				Syringe driver started	

Figure 5.2: STAS chart for Mr T

Could STAS be incorporated into practice?

STAS was incorporated into the teams' work. It took staff between 30 and 90 minutes, at the weekly meetings, to record the scores on all their current patients (10 to 25 patients for each team member). Most time was spent on the assessment of new patients, since the team member would usually discuss this with colleagues. Thereafter, rating a patient who was stable and had been in care for several weeks would take only a minute or two to complete. Twenty STAS ratings (including five first assessments) were timed; the median time to complete a rating was two minutes (range 1 to 15).

Results of audit with STAS

Five teams used the STAS on consecutive patients referred over six months or more. STAS ratings were commenced for 487 patients. For 53 patients (11%), STAS ratings were recorded only at referral, and the patients then died or were discharged before a second assessment was made. Two or more STAS ratings were recorded in the remaining 434 patients (89%): 98 were subsequently discharged and not re-admitted during the study, two died suddenly of diseases other than their cancer, and 334 were in team care at death. Characteristics of the patients referred are shown in Box 5.4.

Box 5.4: Characteristics of patients referred to the teams

487 patients – 54% men and 46% women
Mean age (95% confidence interval) – 66 years (65–67)
Diagnoses – primary cancer of:
  23% lung
  28% gastrointestinal
  18% genitourinary
  10% breast
  4% ear, nose and throat
  4% lymphatic
  7% other
  7% primary tumour not known.
One patient had AIDS and one motor neurone disease.

The percentage of cancer deaths in each area referred to the teams ranged from 23 to 33%.

Missed and late STAS assessments

Assessments for items were sometimes missed, especially 'spiritual' and 'financial' (*see* Table 5.1). Assessments may be missed early in care but then recorded later when teams feel they knew the patient or family well enough to enquire about the problem. Such assessments were defined as 'late assessments' and were common for five STAS items: spiritual, financial, family insight, family anxiety and communication between patient and family. These were assessed late in 20 to 24% of patients. Sometimes items were missed throughout care, and this was common for the item spiritual which was missed throughout care in 50% of patients. For other items, especially pain control and symptom control, there were few missed assessments.

	Assessed late		Missed throughout care	
Item	n	(%)	n	(%)
Pain control	26	(5.3)	2	(0.4)
Symptom control	21	(4.3)	3	(0.6)
Patient anxiety	37	(7.6)	14	(2.9)
Family anxiety	99	(20.3)	50	(10.3)
Patient insight	69	(14.2)	46	(9.5)
Family insight	107	(22.0)	48	(9.9)
Predictability	44	(9.0)	6	(1.2)
Planning	84	(17.3)	34	(7.0)
Practical aid	43	(8.8)	16	(3.3)
Financial	119	(24.4)	81	(16.6)
Wasted time	36	(7.4)	15	(3.1)
Spiritual	109	(22.4)	241	(49.5)
Communication between patient and family	115	(23.6)	58	(11.9)
Communication between professionals	23	(4.7)	7	(1.4)
Communication from professionals to patient and family	43	(8.8)	12	(2.5)
Professional anxiety	19	(3.9)	2	(0.4)
Advising professionals	25	(5.1)	6	(1.2)

Table 5.1: STAS ratings which were assessed late (missed at first contact but then assessed later during care) or were missed throughout care, in the 487 patients included in the audit

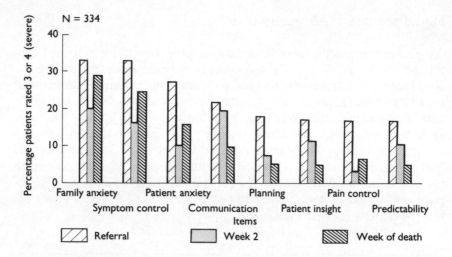

Figure 5.3: Most severe STAS items during care: percentage of patients rated 3 or 4 (severe) during care

Audit of the 334 patients who died in care

The 334 patients spent a mean of 7.8 weeks in care, median five weeks (inter-quartile range two to ten weeks). Figure 5.3 shows the eight most severe items and how the percentage of patients with severe ratings (scores of 3 or 4) changed during care.

(a) At referral
At referral, high proportions (22 to 33%) of patients had severe problems (rated 3 or 4) for four items: family anxiety, symptom control, patient anxiety and communication between patient and family. For another four items: planning, patient insight, pain control and pre-dictability, between 17% and 18% of patients had severe problems (rated 3 or 4). For the remaining nine items (seven concerned with the services, plus spiritual and family insight) there were usually mild problems or none and less than 10% were rated 3 or 4.

(b) Second week of care
By week 2, for all items, fewer patients had severe ratings and more were rated zero (no problems). Compared to ratings at referral, differences were significant for 15 items, all except financial and spiritual (*see* Table 5.2). The four items family anxiety, symptom control, patient anxiety and communication between patient and family

remained relatively severe: 9 to 21% were rated 3 or 4. For other items, 11% or less were rated 3 or 4, and 62 to 97% were rated 0 or 1 (nil or mild problems).

(c) At death

At death, three items: family anxiety, symptom control and patient anxiety continued to be the most severe, and the percentage of patients with severe ratings (score 3 or 4) increased.

| | Wilcoxon matched-pairs signed-ranks test | | | | | |
| | referral v week 2 | | | referral v death | | |
Item	n pairs	Z	p value	n pairs	Z	p value
Pain control	211	−5.94	p<0.00005	241	−5.51	p<0.00005
Symptom control	287	−5.83	p<0.00005	322	−5.34	p<0.00005
Patient anxiety	279	−6.27	p<0.00005	308	−7.06	p<0.00005
Family anxiety	264	−3.42	p=0.0006	294	−2.16	p=0.03
Patient insight	269	−2.24	p=0.03	288	−8.23	p<0.00005
Family insight	260	−2.11	p=0.03	291	−7.61	p<0.00005
Predictability	288	−4.11	p<0.00005	322	−9.91	p<0.00005
Planning	263	−5.18	p<0.00005	304	−8.11	p<0.00005
Practical aid	276	−3.93	p=0.0001	316	−5.59	p<0.00005
Financial	242	−0.85	NS	276	−5.01	p<0.00005
Wasted time	278	−2.50	p=0.01	315	−3.81	p=0.0001
Spiritual	146	−1.19	NS	162	−2.68	p=0.007
Communication between patient and family	249	−3.85	p=0.0001	277	−7.30	p<0.00005
Communication between professionals	287	−3.73	p=0.0002	322	−4.68	p<0.00005
Communication from professionals to patient and family	280	−5.14	p<0.00005	315	−8.11	p<0.00005
Professional anxiety	288	−6.99	p<0.00005	325	−5.73	p<0.00005
Advising professionals	285	−7.95	p<0.00005	319	−7.90	p<0.00005

Table 5.2: Wilcoxon matched-pairs signed-ranks test for referral versus week 2 ratings and for referral versus death ratings. The 334 patients who died in care

Symptom control

The ratings of the item symptom control and the record of a main symptom each week allowed analysis of the changing main symptoms during care. Figure 5.4 shows the eight symptoms (other than pain) most commonly recorded as the main symptom at referral and at death.

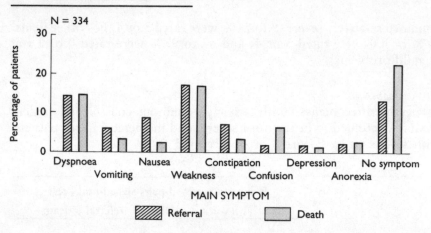

Figure 5.4: Eight most common main symptoms at referral and death (excluding pain)

The most frequent main symptoms were weakness (recorded in 17.1% at referral and 16.7% at death) and dyspnoea (breathlessness – 14.0% at referral and 15.5% at death). Between referral and death, vomiting, nausea and constipation were recorded less frequently as main symptoms, and the number of patients with no symptoms increased. However, confusion became more frequent, and depression and anorexia remained largely unchanged.

The ratings for two common main symptoms dyspnoea, and nausea and vomiting (combined) are shown in Figures 5.5 and 5.6. Teams apparently failed to alleviate dyspnoea, for there was no significant difference between ratings at referral and week 2, death −2 or death. Ratings for nausea and vomiting (combined) were significantly lower in the weeks of death −2 and death compared to referral. The ratings for the item pain control were very different from these two symptoms (*see* Figure 5.7). Ratings had improved markedly by week 2, compared to referral, and this was maintained until death.

Feedback and closing the audit loop

The results suggested the following:

1. The audit was practical and did not intrude into the teams' work too much, although all teams would have liked fewer items.
2. STAS identified aspects which the teams were unable to assess, for example, spiritual needs. This led teams to examine their competence in this area.

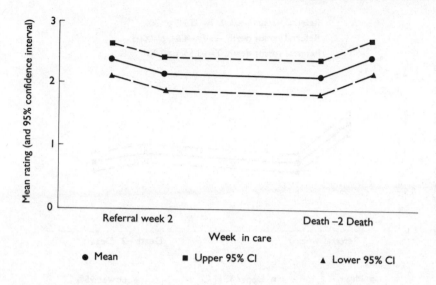

Figure 5.5: Dyspnoea as the main symptom. Mean (95% confidence interval) symptom control rating

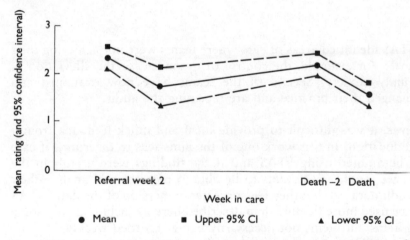

Figure 5.6: Nausea or vomiting as the main symptom. Mean (95% confidence interval) ratings for symptom control. Referral versus death −2, T = −2.54, p = 0.01; Referral versus death, T = −3.61, p = 0.001

3. STAS proved useful in day to day practice, especially for new members of staff, by giving them a check list of important aspects of care which they were not to overlook.
4. STAS identified areas of care where teams were achieving their goals, such as pain control.

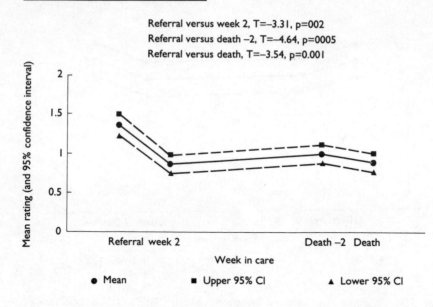

Figure 5.7: Mean (95% confidence interval) ratings for pain control

5. STAS identified areas of care where teams were not achieving their goals, for example, the control of dyspnoea, or the alleviation of family anxiety. Several of the teams have now examined and changed their practice and are repeating the audit.

However, it was difficult to provide local and quick feedback from a central location. In this work one of the aims was to determine if care could be audited using STAS and if the findings were useful. In the future, we would wish teams to be able to monitor and analyse their own audit data, so that they feel a greater ownership of the data. STAS could be used more flexibly than described here by including only some of the items and items not necessarily being recorded weekly.

Adapting STAS for other community services

The Support Team Assessment Schedule can be used to audit other community services which provide palliative care, for example in general practice and district nursing. Here it may be more appropriate to use a few of the items, perhaps only one or two. Chapter 6 discusses the reduction of STAS to nine items which may be used more widely and incorporates the most practical, reliable and valid items.

Conclusions

The Support Team Assesssment Schedule was developed to audit the outcome of community palliative care teams. STAS has 17 items, each graded 0–4, and can be recorded regularly on patients during care. It was developed with and used by five teams caring mainly for patients with cancer, and demonstrated areas where care was effective eg the control of pain, and also where care was less effective eg spiritual assessment and the alleviation of dyspnoea and family anxiety. The results have been fed back to teams and the new practices are being audited.

Acknowledgements

I am grateful to Help the Hospices, who contributed to the funding of this work, and to my colleague Dr Mark McCarthy with whom much of the work was carried out.

References

1 Hospice Information Service (1992) *1992 Directory of Hospice Services in the United Kingdom and Republic of Ireland*. St Christopher's Hospice, 51 Lawrie Park Road, Sydenham, London SE26 6D2.

2 McCarthy M and Higginson IJ (1991) Clinical audit by a palliative care team. *Palliative Medicine* 5(3): 215–221.

3 McKelvie SJ (1978) Graphic rating scales – How many categories? *British Journal of Psychology* 69: 185–202.

6

Audit Methods: Validation and In-patient Use

IRENE HIGGINSON

Introduction

This chapter describes the validation and reliability of the Support Team Assessment Schedule (STAS, *see* Chapter 5) and how STAS can be adapted for in-patient rather than community care.

Validity and reliability are defined in Chapter 3. For STAS various aspects were tested. Mechanisms for adapting STAS included discussion with in-patient hospices about which items were most relevant for their use, and the results of the use of STAS when the patients of support teams had been in hospitals or hospices.

Validity and reliability of STAS

1. Face validity
A scale should yield information of real relevance to the auditor. Methods to assess face validity for STAS are shown in Box 6.1

Box 6.1: Face validity

For STAS, it was agreed that face validity would be satisfied if:

1. STAS items made logical sense to palliative clinicians and could be used in clinical practice.
2. There was a consensus of agreement from clinicians who dealt with dying patients (consensus validity).
3. Clinicians agreed that the range of their work with patients and families was included (content validity).

Face validity was met by, first, presenting STAS at a series of meetings of hospice, hospital, community, and scientific professionals and, second, asking four other support teams, based in southeast England, to test the STAS with their practice for short periods and to comment on and determine if the items reflected their practice.

2. Criterion validity

One main flaw of STAS is that it relies on professional assessments which may be biased, see Chapters 3 and 10. However, the advantage of STAS is that it can be completed on all patients during care. Therefore, we assessed the validity of STAS through comparisons with the views of patients and family members.

STAS ratings completed by two support teams were compared with patients' ratings and family member/carer ratings of seven (of the total 17 STAS) items, collected by independent interviewers. The number of items was limited because patients were unable to complete a lengthy questionnaire interview. Patients' and families' views and comments were also recorded in the questionnaire (shown in full in Appendix I) to assess the quality of care further[1].

Eighty-four patients were interviewed and 67 of these had family members or carers, all of whom were interviewed. Agreement was tested for using Cohen's Kappa, weighted – which shows the proportion of ratings which agree but controls for change agreement. Agreement between team and patient was high for four items, and showed moderate correlations (Spearman's rho ranged $0.45 - 0.66$) for five items, excepting two items including family needs (see Box 6.2). The summed scores for seven items were correlated, Spearman's rho $= 0.66$, $p < 0.0001$. Where differences were found team members identified more problems than patients' self-ratings, except for one item, pain control, where team members identified fewer problems. Team ratings were usually closer to those of patients than to those of family members, and often lay between the patient and family member ratings[2].

Further testing of validity involved comparing STAS with a previously validated quality of life measure – the Hebrew Rehabilitation Centre for the Aged Quality of Life Index (HRCA-QL) which was used in the United States National Hospice Study. The HRCA-QL has five items: health, daily living, mobility, support and outlook, each rated $0-2$[3]. We found reasonable correlations between items which were similar, for example, symptom control (STAS) with health (HRCA-QL) Spearman rho $= -0.64$, or patient anxiety (STAS) with outlook (HRCA-QL) Spearman rho $= -0.70$, both $p < 0.0005$[4]. However, correlations were highest in patients seen more than four weeks before death and were low near death. Near death most patients had very low scores on the HRCA-QL.

Box 6.2

Team versus patient ratings. The proportion of ratings which were equal or within one score; the proportion where of ratings were different; the weighted kappas; and correlation coefficients.

Item	number of pairs	Ratings equal or +1 or −1	Proportion of pairs		Weighted Kappa	Spearman rho	Patient mean (SD)
			Team rating <patient ratings −1	Team rating >patient rating +1			
Pain control	66	0.97	0.03	0	0.53	0.66#*	1.14 (1.04)
Symptom control	76	0.91	0.05	0.04	0.40	0.59#*	1.59 (1.09)
Patient anxiety	76	0.87	0.03	0.11	0.28	0.45#*	0.73 (1.01)
Family anxiety	62	0.77	0.11	0.11	0.12	0.26*	1.60 (1.28)
Practical	76	0.99	0	0.01	0.78	0.78#*	0.10 (0.31)
Wasted time	78	0.96	0.01	0.01	0.48	0.49#*	0.10 (0.42)
Communication of professionals to patient and family	74	0.89	0	0.11	0.08	0.18	0.05 (0.31)

* $p < 0.05$ #* $p < 0.0001$

Team versus family member ratings. The proportion of ratings which were equal or within one score; the proportion where of ratings were different; the weighted kappas; and correlation coefficients.

Item	number of pairs	Ratings equal or +1 or −1	Proportion of pairs		Weighted Kappa	Spearman rho
			Team rating <FM ratings −1	Team rating >FM rating +1		
Pain control	58	0.84	0.16	0	0.42	0.66#*
Symptom control	66	0.76	0.24	0	0.13	0.21*
Patient anxiety	65	0.74	0.22	0.05	0.18	0.31**
Family anxiety	66	0.74	0.21	0.05	0.15	0.20$
Practical	67	0.99	0	0.01	0.51	0.42#
Wasted time	67	0.91	0.04	0.04	−0.06	−0.09
Communication of professionals to patient and family	63	0.92	0.02	0.06	0.23	0.27*

* $p < 0.05$ ** $p < 0.01$ # $p < 0.001$ #* $p < 0.0001$
$ $p = 0.05$

3. Reliability

To enhance the reliability of STAS ratings, definitions and gradings for each STAS item were provided to each team member in their own individual booklet for use while making assessments. Team members were also trained in the use of STAS ratings before commencing the audit and were encouraged to discuss difficulties.

To test the reliability of STAS, team members completed assessments on 45 patients and their ratings were compared. It was not practical for members of the same team to visit the same patients simultaneously, and it was clearly impossible for members of different teams to assess the same patients at the same time. Therefore, written descriptions of patients (simulated patients) abstracted from team notes and the weekly meetings were used.

The second test of reliability was to measure the internal consistency of STAS statistically. The results of the reliability testing are shown in Box 6.3.

The results of the validity testing indicated that STAS was a reasonable measure and reflected the views of patients and families, although the teams' ratings did not agree completely. STAS also correlated with a quality of life measure. However, we were not able to test all the STAS items. One item, predictability, proved unreliable. These results were considered when suggesting a shortened STAS for in-patient use.

Amendments made to items included in STAS

Through discussion with the in-patient units and the teams about STAS it was agreed that there were nine core items which were most relevant to in-patient care. This omitted those items which were related to the advisory nature of support teams; those items which had been shown to be least reliable and valid in testing; those items which were often missed (eg spiritual); and those items related to service provision in the

---

Box 6.3: Results of reliability of STAS

Test-retest: 45 patients each with two to nine assessors
For 16 out of 17 items ratings were equal or $+1/-1$ score for 88% or more of the cases. There were highly significant ($p < 0.0005$) Cohen's Kappas, $0.48-0.87$ and high correlation coefficients (Spearman's rho ranged $0.65-0.94$, $p < 0.0005$). One item, predictability, did not reach our pre-set standards. Where missed assessments were recorded, the pairs commonly agreed on a missed assessment.

Internal consistency
Tests of internal consistency included Spearman Brown split half reliability and Cronbach's alpha. Coefficients ranged $0.68-0.89$[4].

For Cohen's Kappa, Spearman correlations, Spearman Brown and Cronbach's alpha a coefficient of $0 = $ worst, $1 = $ best possible.

community, such as practical aid and wasted time. However, if patients were admitted for respite or were to be discharged these items might then be considered. It was also agreed that the definition of symptoms might need to be expanded because patients were often admitted for symptom control. This has been carried out, *see* Chapter 14. The core nine items are shown in Box 6.4, the definitions of STAS are as shown in Appendix A.

Box 6.4: The nine core STAS items

Pain control
Symptom control
Patient anxiety
Patient insight
Family anxiety
Family insight
Communication between patient and family
Communication from professionals to patient and family
Communication between professionals

The items patient insight and family insight are included although these are not truly goals of care. Palliative care staff will create opportunities to openly discuss prognosis and diagnosis, but do not necessarily seek to change insight if a patient indicates they do not wish to change. However, most staff felt that they wished to record these items for clinical use even if they would not intervene.

Amendments to the frequency of ratings

In the support teams STAS ratings had been recorded at referral and then weekly until death or discharge. This was appropriate for community based teams where the median time in care was seven weeks. However, in-patients were frequently admitted for shorter periods, often as short as two weeks. Also their condition fluctuated considerably. In hospital and in hospice it proved more difficult to average the patient's condition over the previous one week. Therefore STAS recordings may need to be made more frequently, perhaps twice a week.

Other amendments

The ideal standard for each item was a score of zero. This could be achieved for some items, but clearly not all. It may be that teams would wish to set more realistic standards for some items. For example, a possible standard for family anxiety might be that less than 20% of families have ratings which are severe at death.

Other limitations and ways forward

STAS includes 17 items across a wide range of palliative care, but detailed information on each item, for example the type of pain, is not included. In particular, the psychological and social aspects of STAS are rudimentary, and it appears from the results that depression is under-reported[4]. Other psychological aspects, such as anger, loss, fear, shock, withdrawal, guilt, confusion and anticipatory grief, also occur in terminal cancer[5], but are not measured by STAS. STAS reflects only the patient- and family-orientated work of support teams, but not their other work, including bereavement care, formal education of other health professionals, and self-management of their service. There is clearly a need for the development of better measures in all of these areas. However, it is also important to be practical – the number of aspects which can reliably and usefully be recorded on patients at any one time is limited. It would be a disaster for patient care if professionals became subsumed in recording every possible aspect of care. Perhaps a useful way forward is for professionals to test and use some of the most reliable and valid measures available for fairly short periods, attempting to complete the audit cycle and improve care and then move on to audit other aspects.

Conclusions

STAS was found to have measurable validity and reliability through a series of studies which compared staff ratings with those made independently by patients and their family members, compared STAS with a quality of life index, and compared different raters. Through further discussion with in-patient staff STAS was shortened to nine items, and the frequency of assessments was varied.

Acknowledgements

I am grateful to Help the Hospices, who contributed to the funding of this work, and to my colleague Dr Mark McCarthy with whom much of the work was carried out.

References

1 Higginson I, Wade A and McCarthy M (1990) Palliative care: views of patients and their families. *British Medical Journal* **301**: 277–81.

2 Higginson I and McCarthy M (1993) Validity of the Support Team Assessment Schedule: do staffs' ratings reflect those made by patients and their families? *Palliative Medicine* **7**: 219–28.

3 Greer DS, Mor V, Morris JN, Sherwood S, Kidder D and Birnbaum H (1986) An alternative in terminal care: results of the National Hospice Study. *Journal of Chronic Disease* **39**: 9–26.

4 Higginson I (1992) *The development, validity, reliability and practicality of a new measure of palliative care – the Support Team Assessment Schedule*. PhD Thesis. University of London.

5 Cassidy S (1986) Emotional distress in terminal cancer: discussion paper. *Journal of the Royal Society of Medicine* **79**: 717–20.

Further reading

Streiner DL and Norman GR (1989) *Health measurement scales. A practical guide to their development and use*. Oxford: Oxford University Press.

7

Audit Methods: Regional Documentation Standards

ROBERT A CATTERALL*

Introduction

With the recent changes in the working of the NHS, more attention is being focused on audit and monitoring. In the palliative and continuing care areas this is particularly so and pressures are being brought to bear on all of us to demonstrate the performance of our contracts in terms of the quality of care given as well as the quantity of care.

Monitoring the performance of care in relation to the quality of life is more difficult than monitoring the curative process of disease due principally to the difficulty in defining 'quality of life'[1,2,3]. Hospice units are often small and widely dispersed so that medical audit by a peer group can be a problem. We therefore came together on a regional basis. Initially five units in the Trent Region agreed to work together, with the objectives shown in Box 7.1. Taking a lead from the Royal

*On behalf of Trent Hospice Audit Group

Mr John Hunt, Nightingale Macmillan Continuing Care Unit
Mrs Jean Freeman, Ashgate Hospice
Mrs Margaret Carradice, St Luke's Hospice
Mrs Bronwyn Biswas, Leicestershire Hospice
Dr Tony Crowther, St Luke's Hospice
Mrs Margaret Duffy, Staunton Harold Hospice
Dr G Rathbone, Staunton Harold Hospice

Dr Joanna Hocknall, Nottingham Hospice
Dr Vaughan Keeley, Macmillan Continuing Care Unit
Mrs Penny McFaul, St Barnabas' Hospice
Dr Sam Ahmedzai, Leicestershire Hospice
Dr Richard Atkinson, Ashgate Hospice

College of Physicians, we began with audit of patient notes. As we progressed, it became clear that particularly in the hospice setting, team audit would be more appropriate and nursing staff became part of the group[1,2]. The need to restrict the size of the group precluded the co-opting of other team members at this stage. Our nursing colleagues had already begun to develop 'core standards' of hospice care and brought these with them. The core standards became a joint project (*see* Chapter 9).

Box 7.1: Objectives

● Regional hospice audit.
● Establish standards and audit tools.
● Complete the audit cycle by reviewing clinical practice and standards[4].

Method

Initially the medical directors from five hospices in the Trent Region made a commitment to meet once a month at the most convenient central site. A provisional audit form was devised along the lines of the Royal College of Physicians' paper[5,6,7] to facilitate the extraction of data from the notes. Five sets of case notes were taken from the files at random and given to another colleague to review, noting the results on the audit form[8,9]. We then had an audit review meeting to discuss the results which were presented confidentially with no reference to a particular unit. Later we found that the units preferred to be more open[10].

These results enabled the group to set out a draft copy of documentation standards. These were discussed and refined at several meetings, producing the final draft shown in Appendix D. We began to discuss the core standards and at this time a sixth hospice joined our audit group. At the same time the audit tool to be used in the review of patient notes was revised and the cycle repeated[11].

Results

There were several initial runs using an early audit form. The procedure for bereavement follow-up was deleted from the later audit forms as it was thought this would be better dealt with in a separate audit of the bereavement service. A significant finding of these audits was the recognition of the ways hospices recorded information across medical, nursing and paramedical notes. For example, discussion with the relatives may be noted in the nursing notes but not in medical notes. Information was taken from various sources as required and did not need to be duplicated. This increased our awareness of the need for 'team' audit rather than medical audit. We therefore agreed that information was to be regarded as recorded, regardless of where in the notes it came from, and auditing was not to be restricted to the doctors' notes.

Having formed a more structured approach to the notes it was more easily recognized that we had missed out important information areas. The group now felt confident enough to write documentation standards. After an initial draft and much discussion we established our standards (Appendix E) and wrote a new audit tool to review notes against these standards (Appendix F). A computer program was created (apply to Dr Robert Catterall, Medical Director, St Barnabas' Hospice, 36 Nettleham Road, Lincoln LN2 1RE for further information) to collate and review the results in a standardized form, presenting them without reference to individual units.

Appendix G shows the detailed results of one unit (under a code name) and Figure 7.1 shows the overall results of all the units. We still found that some questions were misleading or irrelevant. For example 'special instructions to relatives' may not have been noted because there were no relatives. Later we determined that where such information was thought to be sufficiently important to be part of the standard, its absence should be noted. From the results it can be seen that ethnic origin was often missed out despite several of our hospices being located in areas with sizeable populations of differing ethnic groups. Time of admission and of medical assessment was often incomplete, making any

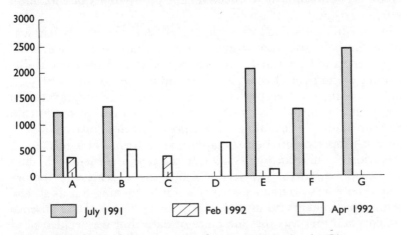

Figure 7.1: Sum of the per cent of omissions (units A–G)

audit of delay difficult. Surprisingly, occupation was often missing or difficult to find unless the patient had mesothelioma. As a result of this, one of the hospices has introduced a barrier in their computer clinical database program that forces entry of at least 'cancer related' or 'not cancer related' occupation, including a reminder if the primary diagnosis is known to be related to certain occupations.

At the end of the computer printout of the results of a single unit's audit, a list shows the percentage of notes not recording particular items of data. Adding the percentage omission figures for each unit (Figure 7.1) shows a significant drop from 1991 (when it ranged from 1324 to 2460) to 1992 (when it ranged from 124 to 657).

Discussion

From the first meeting it became clear that our assumption that we all did more or less the same things was false. Documentation at each hospice however was not sufficiently different to prevent the development of documentation standards. Bereavement notes were soon seen to be sufficiently different for a separate audit to be more appropriate. The early recognition of the need for team audit helped us to revise both the standards and the audit tool. It became clear that the documentation needed to be taken as a whole, that is medical, nursing and paramedical notes, especially in relation to communication with the patient and relatives[12].

The combination of audit of notes and review meeting worked well to begin with. However, later discussion of standards and audit took all the available time for the meeting so that audit of the notes had to be done separately. This indicated a need for the group to acquire an audit facilitator.

The documentation standards included all that the group felt was essential in the palliative care situation rather than all that we could reasonably expect to be entered. It was expected that in the early audits there would be a number of omissions. As can be seen from the results, the number of these omissions was far greater than expected. On investigation it was found that most tasks had been completed but no note had been made. For example, all the post discharge tasks had been done but not properly noted on the appropriate form. This has led to reconsideration of the recording system. In the case of patients who had a pacemaker fitted, there is a need for this to be dealt with before cremation. There was no incidence of this not happening but as so few patients have pacemakers no unit regularly made a note of the absence of pacemaker and this was the one piece of data that we decided need not be entered in every patient's notes. In the other areas of missing data this necessitated drawing it to the attention of the staff and in some cases reorganizing the system and form of documentation.

Several of the group suggested that an alternative to 'no note' would be useful and we have again added a 'not adequate' to the audit tool. At present it is proposed to use this only as an aid to finding the reason for missing data but the routine reports on the audits at present only register data as present or absent.

Reports of the results of audit need to be easily read and assimilated. In order to produce these and standardize them a computer program was written, the results of which can be seen in Appendix G. From these reports it is easy to see where the omissions were made and the overall percentages of omissions so that comparisons can be made in succeeding audits.

Core standards have been produced and published. Little can be said about the core standards at this stage because they have not been subject to proper detailed testing. However, they do represent the consensus view of the region's in-patient hospice directors of nursing services and medical directors. Their development is reviewed in Chapter 9.

Producing audit tools that are seen to be both appropriate and educational (that is leading to improvement in or better recognition of care needed) with minimal interference in day to day work should be our goal. Tips to help the development of audit are shown in Box 7.2.

Box 7.2: Tips

- The team should meet on a regional basis.
- Decide what to audit.
- Develop the tools.
- Let the team examine the results.
- Examination of results may lead to a change in the ways of working.
- Repeat the audit.

References

1 Hockley JM, Dunlop R and Davies RJ (1988) Survey of distressing symptoms in dying patients and their families in hospital and the response to a symptom control team. *British Medical Journal* **296:** 1715–17.

2 Royal College of Physicians (1991) *Palliative care: guidelines for good practice and audit measures.*

3 SCOPME (1989) *Medical audit and the educational implications.* Standing Committee on Postgraduate Medical Education.

4 Gabbay J, McNicol M, Spilby J, Davies S and Layton AJ (1990) What did audit achieve? Lessons from preliminary evaluation of a year's medical audit. *British Medical Journal* **301**: 526–9.

5 Ellis BW (1988) How to set up an audit. *British Medical Journal* **298**: 1635–7.

6 Royal College of Physicians (1989) *Medical audit, a first report. What, why and how.* London: Royal College of Physicians.

7 Shaw C (1989) *Medical audit. A hospital handbook.* London: King's Fund Centre FC89/11.

8 Bennett J and Shaw CD (1988) *Guidance on what should be in the clinical medical records for the Brighton Health District.* Brighton District Health Authority, 103–9.

9 Ellis BW and Sensky T (1991) A clinician's guide to setting up audit. *British Medical Journal* **302**: 704–7.

10 Walshe K and Bennett J (1991) *Guidelines on medical audit and confidentiality.* South East Thames RHA.

11 Smith T (1990) Medical audit. *British Medical Journal* **300**: 65.

12 Blyth AC (1990) Audit of terminal care in general practice. *British Medical Journal* **300**: 983–6.

Further reading

Clinical Resource and Audit Group (1990) Confidentiality and medical audit – interim guidelines, Sept. Scottish Home and Health Dept.

Trent Region Hospice Audit Group (1992) *Palliative care core standards.* Derby: Nightingale Macmillan Unit.

8

Audit Methods: The Edmonton Symptom Assessment System

EDUARDO BRUERA AND SUSAN MACDONALD

Introduction

More than 50% of patients with a diagnosis of cancer will die of advanced disease[1]. Most advanced cancer patients suffer from a variety of devastating symptom complexes[2,3,4]. A number of sophisticated assessment systems have been developed for pain[5-7], dyspnoea[8], nausea[9,10] and psychological symptoms[11-13].

Each of these instruments have been validated and are reliable for the assessment and follow-up of different patient populations. Some instruments are complete but very lengthy and/or require training prior to implementation, while others are simple and suitable for repetition.

The current delivery of medical care requires various physicians, nurses, and other disciplines to treat a given patient over time. Therefore, a system that would allow for a rapid assessment of different symptoms and for fast interpretation of the results might be beneficial to the continuity of patient care. The tool would need to be easily interpreted by all health care providers and be capable of being implemented by any member of the team at any given time. A graphic display of information has proven to be highly effective in the interpretation of the variables such as blood pressure, temperature or sequential neurological examination and would be a desirable feature.

Because of the absence of such a tool for the assessment of multiple symptoms, we designed the Edmonton Symptom Assessment System (ESAS). The purpose of this chapter is to describe our experience during the development and testing of the ESAS in a population of advanced cancer patients.

Description of the Edmonton Symptom Assessment System (ESAS)

Patients are usually considered to be the best judges of the symptoms they experience. By utilizing their assessments repeatedly, values are rated against their own controls. A tool which is simple and rapidly completed ensures that even debilitated, terminally ill patients can comply. While there are many methods of assessments[5,9,11,12] visual analogue scales (VAS) are quite simple and effective tools. These have now been validated by clinical trials[7].

The Edmonton Symptom Assessment System (ESAS) tool itself consists of nine visual analogue scales. These include pain, shortness of breath, nausea, depression, activity, anxiety, well-being, drowsiness and appetite (see Figure 8.1). The patient is to draw a mark along the 100 mm line of the VAS. The left side of the line indicates the least degree of symptoms, and the right side indicates the worst symptoms. The patient is asked to correlate his or her assessment of that symptom over the last several hours and place a mark on the line that reflects their assessment. The ESAS is completed twice daily at 10.00 am and 6.00 pm. The patient may complete their VAS scales alone or with the assistance of a nurse depending upon their ability. This takes only a few minutes to complete. Patients who are unable to respond due to cognitive failure, are assessed by their nurse or a specially trained family member. The VAS scales are then converted into numerical form by measuring from the left margin of the line in millimetres to the mark that has been made by the patient. The score out of 100 is then transferred to a bar graph and recorded twice daily (see Figure 8.2). The symptom assessment graph records up to 20 days of values, allowing the staff to visualize patterns of symptom control easily over time. A quick and reliable reference to symptom status can be made at a glance by all members of the health care team. All patients have an ESAS completed on their admission to hospital, and twice daily thereafter.

Space is provided on the symptom assessment sheet for an extra VAS scale. This can be used to record a less frequent symptom particular to an individual patient (eg hiccups, cough, pruritus). The intensity of this symptom would also be assessed twice daily.

The symptom assessment graph contains other information in addition to the symptom profile. Under each day's data, there is space to identify the assessor. Space is also provided for recording the minimental state examination score. This is a simple, 30 item questionnaire that assesses the patient's cognitive function[11]. Correlation can be easily made between symptom profile and the mental status of the patient. The symptom assessment graph is kept on the patient's chart and is available for ongoing review.

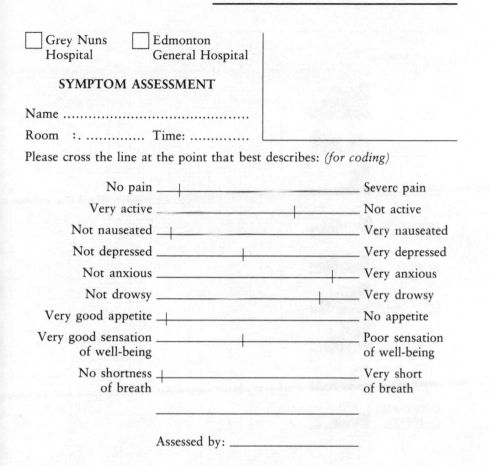

Figure 8.1: Visual analogue scale

Results in cancer patients

In order to determine the effectiveness and usability of this tool, 101 consecutive patients admitted to the Palliative Care Unit, Edmonton General Hospital, were assessed using the ESAS. Patient characteristics are summarized in Table 8.1. A total of 63 052 assessments were carried out during 33 052 patient days for 101 patients. Of these, 85 patients were able to complete their ESAS either alone or assisted by a nurse at admission (84%). As disease progressed, 84/101 patients could not complete the form and it was completed by the nurse in 96% of cases and a relative in 4% of cases. No patient consistently refused to complete the form. Occasionally, patients refused to complete the form on a given day due to tiredness or severe symptoms. In that event, the

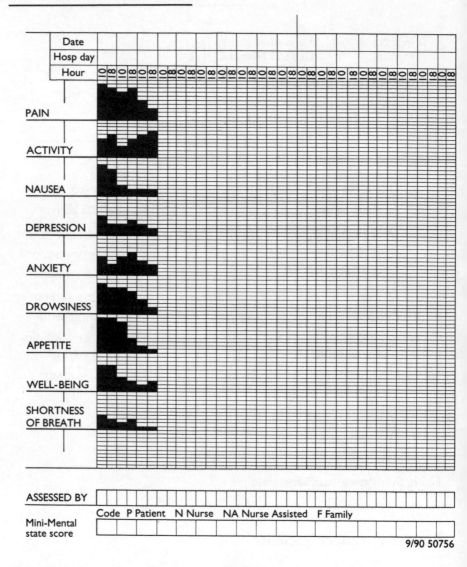

Figure 8.2: Symptom assessment graph

nurse would complete the form for that day and the patient would restart on the following day. By summing the scores of the different variables, we determined a symptom distress score. The highest potential value was 100 mm for each of the nine variables, for a total of 900. Table 8.2 summarizes the mean (and standard deviation) symptom distress score for the first five days of admission of our patients. Scores for day 5 were significantly lower than for day 1.

This initial prospective study suggested that the ESAS could be completed by the majority of our extremely debilitated and symptomatic

Characteristics	Sex (women/men)	57/44
	Mean (and standard deviation) age in years	65 (13)
	Mean (and standard deviation) length of stay in days	34 (36)
Primary tumour	Breast	15
	Genitourinary	20
	Lung	30
	Gastrointestinal	23
	Haematological	3
	Melanoma	3
	Head and neck	6
	Unknown	1
	Total	101

Table 8.1: Patient characteristics

Day after admission	Mean (SD) symptom distress score	Number of patients
Day 1	410 (95*)	101
Day 2	377 (87)	101
Day 3	367 (97)	97
Day 4	374 (73)	95
Day 5	362 (83*)	95

* $P < 0.01$ (student's paired T-test).

Table 8.2: ESAS during first five days of admission

patients. Table 8.2 shows that there was a significant improvement in symptom distress during the first five days of admission, probably as a result of both symptomatic interventions by medical and nursing staff and adjustment by patients to the unit.

Validity and reliability of ESAS

To validate ESAS a second study was undertaken in which we assessed 34 consecutive patients with ESAS twice during the period of one hour, and these results were compared by an assessment performed using the Support Team Assessment Schedule (STAS) (*see* Chapter 5). The STAS was completed by the patient with the assistance of a nurse. Table 8.3 shows the correlation between the ESAS repeated within one hour by the nurse. At the time of their second assessment, 29/34 patients (85%) said they had either scored the same (n = 17) or did not remember (n = 12) as an hour before. One hour after the initial assessment, one patient stated that he felt much worse (3%), eight patients felt worse (23%), 15 patients felt the same (43%), 11 patients felt better (31%), and no patients felt much better (0%). Therefore, 33/34 patients (97%) felt minor or no change in their symptoms.

Table 8.4 summarizes the mean intensity of different symptoms during the first and second assessments. No significant differences were observed.

Table 8.5 summarizes the correlation between ESAS and STAS during the second assessment. With the exception of activity, a very high correlation was found for each of the remaining variables. The second study suggests that different observers did not appear to influence the patients' assessment and that high correlations were observed between the ESAS and STAS over time.

Although more research is needed in order to better define the accuracy of the ESAS in patients with cognitive failure, language, illiteracy or neurological deficits, our results in this sample of cognitively aware patients suggests that ESAS has an acceptable level of validity and reliability.

Symptom	r	p
Pain	0.9	<0.001
Activity	0.5	<0.001
Nausea	0.8	<0.001
Depression	0.8	<0.001
Anxiety	0.8	<0.001
Drowsiness	0.8	<0.001
Appetite	0.9	<0.001
Sensation of well-being	0.6	<0.001
Dyspnoea	0.8	<0.001
SDS*	0.9	<0.001

* Symptom Distress Score (summed score of all items).

Table 8.3: Correlation between different assessments: ESAS first nurse assessment versus second nurse assessment (n = 34)

Symptom	First assessment (mean SD)	P**	Second assessment (mean SD)
Pain	40.3 (27.8)	NS	41.0 (29.6)
Activity	69.2 (26.6)	NS	72.7 (27.9)
Nausea	28.0 (34.4)	NS	23.8 (32.0)
Depression	26.3 (27.7)	NS	25.4 (29.3)
Anxiety	26.9 (27.7)	NS	27.2 (27.0)
Drowsiness	42.2 (35.8)	NS	46.4 (35.6)
Appetite	57.7 (34.9)	NS	52.7 (35.7)
Sensation of well-being	57.1 (26.9)	NS	51.8 (36.7)
Dyspnoea	17.4 (19.1)	NS	15.2 (21.3)
SDS*	367.5 (142.7)	NS	356.0 (155.5)

* Symptom Distress Score (summed score of all items).
** Mean difference between first and second assessment analysed by paired T-test.

Table 8.4: Mean (and standard deviation) ESAS symptom score for first and second assessments

Symptom	r	p
Pain	0.9	<0.001
Activity	0.2	NS
Nausea	0.9	<0.001
Depression	0.7	<0.001
Anxiety	0.8	<0.001
Drowsiness	0.8	<0.001
Appetite	0.8	<0.001
Sensation of well-being	0.8	<0.001
Dyspnoea	0.8	<0.001
SDS*	0.8	<0.0001

* Symptom Distress Score (summed score of all items).

Table 8.5: Correlation between ESAS and STAS on second assessment

Uses of the ESAS

In the following paragraphs, we will describe some of the practical applications of a system like ESAS in a palliative care programme.

Co-ordination of care between different physicians and other disciplines

The necessary fragmentation of care to multiple health professionals sometimes makes continuity of care difficult to maintain. The presence of ESAS scores makes it very simple for physicians or nurses on call and for members of other disciplines to update themselves on the symptom profile of a given patient. A simplified version of the ESAS is regularly used in communication between the palliative care unit, the pain and symptom control clinic at the regional cancer centre, and various family physicians and home care nurses. The use of a standard method of symptom assessment allows community and referral institutions to speak a common language and monitor therapeutic interventions accordingly.

Quality control

The baseline assessment provides a measure of the severity of symptom distress in patients admitted to the palliative care programme. Follow-up assessments measured during regular intervals allow the staff to determine the effectiveness of different treatment interventions. The consequence of a change in the patterns of care can be monitored quite effectively. Patients consistently in good symptom control need to be quickly assessed for discharge planning (*see* Figure 8.3) while patients who die in poor symptom control require a review in order to establish possible causes and to plan for future similar cases (*see* Figure 8.4).

Education and research

Education of physicians and other disciplines is helped by the presence of an ongoing assessment system. Students who need to quickly become familiar with many patients may use the ESAS to follow the course of various symptom complexes, and to understand the relationship between different symptoms. The preparation of teaching rounds and case reports is greatly assisted by the availability of accurate data[14-17].

The interaction between different symptoms in a given patient can allow for a better diagnosis of different symptom problems. Boxes 8.1 to 8.3 summarize three useful cases where reviewing the ESAS proved helpful in understanding the patient's condition or reaction to treatment.

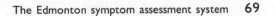

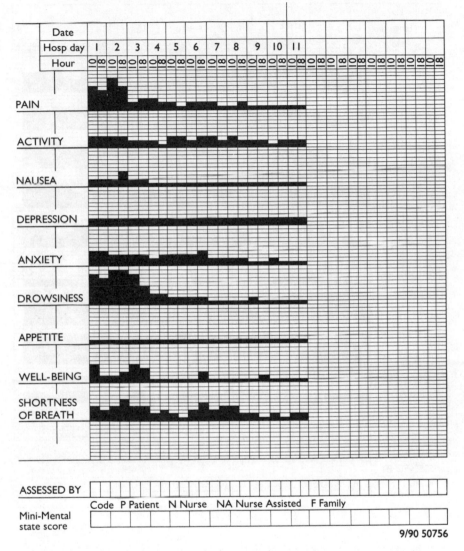

Figure 8.3: Visual analogue scale demonstrating good symptom control

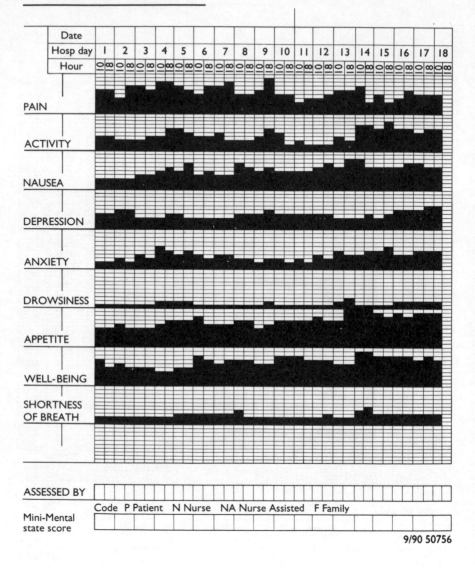

Figure 8.4: Visual analogue scale demonstrating poor symptom control

Box 8.1: Case 1

A 63-year-old female patient with advanced chordoma of the sacrum was admitted with severe pain. Figure 8.5 shows that several increases in opioids did not result in significant analgesia, but did significantly increase sedation and nausea. After three different opioids had been used and a number of adjuvant drugs had been tried, the patient underwent percutaneous cordotomy during day 14. The patient had experienced immediate relief in the main pain syndrome in her left hemipelvis and her left leg. Over the next few days, the dose of opioids and methylphenidate were significantly reduced allowing for a decrease in her level of nausea and sedation.

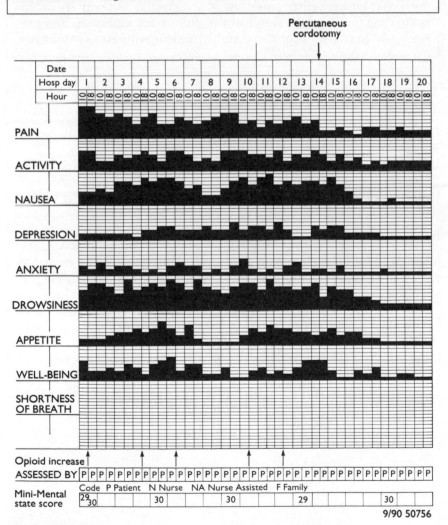

Figure 8.5: VAS: case 1 percutaneous cordotomy on day 14

Box 8.2: Case 2

A 64-year-old woman with advanced carcinoma of the breast with multiple bone metastases was admitted because of poor control of pain and nausea (*see* Figure 8.6). After an increase in the dose of morphine and the institution of both metoclopramide and dexamethasone, good pain control was achieved. Unfortunately, during day 7, she presented with sudden onset of severe dyspnoea and chest pain. The diagnosis of pulmonary embolism was made and oxygen, subcutaneous heparin, and an increase in the dose of morphine were administered. Her dyspnoea progressively improved over the next few days. Her appetite, sensation of well-being, and activity deteriorated significantly as a result of the pulmonary embolism and progressively improved after successful treatment with anti-coagulation.

Box 8.3: Case 3

A 54-year-old man with advanced non-small cell carcinoma of the lung with multiple bony and lung metastases was admitted complaining of a large number of symptoms (*see* Figure 8.7). The pattern of extreme severity in most symptoms with low levels of anxiety and depression had previously suggested to us the presence of somatization. This patient required high doses of opioids on an unpredictable basis and for an unclear pain syndrome. Although initially denied by the patient and the family, it later became clear that the patient had a history of heavy alcohol intake and was used to dealing with stress by consuming alcohol. During day 11, the patient was confronted with this coping mechanism and intensive counselling by the staff including psychology, nursing, social work and pastoral care was started. Over the next few days there was a significant decrease in the generalized complaint of symptoms and it was possible to decrease the opioid intake from a mean equivalent daily dose of 2800 mg of morphine a day to a total of 300 mg of morphine a day.

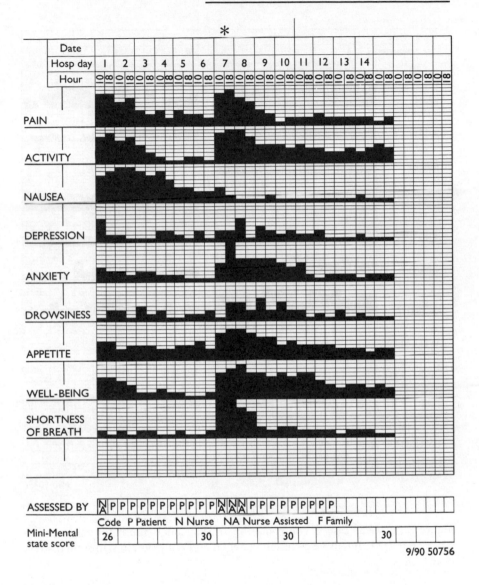

Figure 8.6: VAS: case 2 initial response to therapy noted. *Pulmonary embolism on day 7

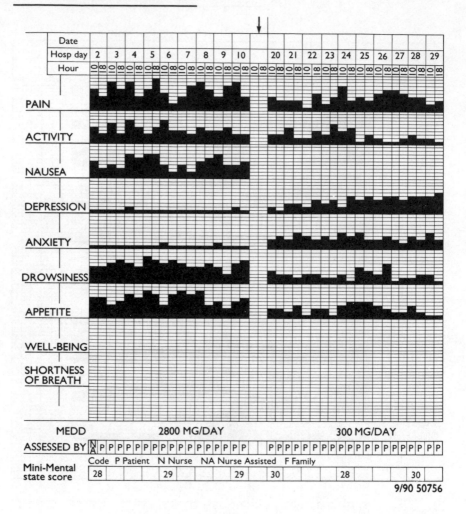

Figure 8.7: VAS: case 3 confrontation of substance abuse for coping with stress on day 11. Intensive counselling begun and reduction in symptom distress noted

The ESAS allowed us to have an idea of the patient's perception in these three clinical situations and also provided us with a measure of the relative success of our therapeutic interventions.

Future work

The reliability of the ESAS should be better established in a number of patient populations. In several groups of patients, including illiterate or non-English speaking patients, or those impaired by significant cognitive or affective disorders, the ESAS has not been adequately validated. The visual analogue scale could be replaced in some of these populations by verbal descriptors, numbers, or even drawings of objects of different sizes.

The correlation between the different symptoms and the relevance of each of these on the patients overall sensation of well-being need to be better established. The effect of somatization syndromes and addiction on symptom profiles should also be evaluated. The effect of successful management of some symptom complexes on the intensity of other symptom complexes should also be a focus of future research.

The validity of the assessments performed by a third person (such as the nurse or a family member) should be better established. Initial work by MacEachern did show some significant correlations between nurse and patient for symptoms such as dyspnoea and depression (correlations ranged 0.3 to 0.3)[18]. However, their assessments of sensation of well-being were not correlated, and the degree of correlation varied during care. Also, the frequency of assessments should be reviewed. While very unstable patients might require assessment more frequently than twice a day, chronically stable patients might require assessment once a day or even less frequently.

Very significant variables such as the overall opiate dose, the functional performance of the patient, and the level of social support are currently not being assessed by the ESAS. Other methods such as the STAS regularly measure some of these variables (*see* Chapter 5). A comprehensive functional assessment of the patient is currently being developed by our group.

Conclusions

The ESAS is a simple and effective test for the baseline and subsequent assessment of symptoms in patients with advanced cancer. It has the advantage of standardizing data, which facilitates communication among health care workers. It has been proven to be easily completed by debilitated cancer patients and to be reliable when a third party completes the assessment for the patient. Periodic review of the ESAS permits the recognition of symptom patterns and responses to interventions. This information is useful in both research studies and at the bedside.

Further studies are required to validate the usefulness of the ESAS in a variety of patient populations. It is likely that, with ongoing evaluation, the final instrument will undergo significant changes. However, it is clear that the principle of standardized symptom assessments by a tool such as the ESAS, has value in clinical use.

References

1 World Health Organisation Expert Committee (1990) *Cancer pain relief*, palliative care report of the WHO Expert Committee, Geneva, Switzerland: World Health Organisation: 12.

2 Baines M (1978) Control of other symptoms. In: Saunders CM (ed.) *The management of terminal disease*. Chicago: Yearbook.

3 Billings JA (1985) The management of common symptoms. In: Billings JA (ed.) *Outpatient management of advanced cancer*. Philadelphia: JB Lippincott: 41.

4 Bruera E (1990) Symptom control in patients with cancer. *Journal of Psychosocial Oncology* 8(2/3): 47–73.

5 Bruera E, Macmillan K, Hanson J and MacDonald RN (1989) The Edmonton staging system for cancer pain: preliminary report. *Pain* 37: 203–9.

6 Melzack R (1975) The McGill pain questionnaire: major properties and scoring methods. *Pain* 1: 277–99.

7 Price DD, McGrath P and Rafti A. *et al*. (1983) The validation of a visual analog scale or ratio scale for pain. *Pain* 17: 45–6.

8 Mahler D, Weinberg D and Wells C *et al*. (1984) The measurement of dyspnoea. *Chest* 85: 751–8.

9 Bruera E, Cowan L, Chadwick S, Drebit D, Hanson J, MacDonald RN and van Konkelenberg Y (1986) Caloric intake assessment in advanced cancer patients: a comparison of three methods. *Cancer Treatment Reports* 70(8): 981–3.

10 Venner P, Bruera E, Drebit D and Shankowsky H (1986) Intensive treatment scheduling of nabilone plus dexamethasone vs metoclopramide plus dexamethasone in cisplatinum-induced emesis. *Proceedings of the American Society of Clinical Oncology* 5(988): 253.

11 Folstein MF, Folstein SE and McHugh PR (1975) 'Mini mental state': a practical method for grading the cognitive state of patients for the clinician. *Journal of Psychiatric Research* 12: 189–98.

12 Tomb DA (1988) *Psychiatry for the house officer*. Baltimore: Williams and Wilkins, 12–13.

13 Trzepac PT, Baker RW and Greenhouse J (1988) A symptom rating scale for delirium. *Psychiatry Research* **23**: 89–97.

14 Bruera E, Schoeller T, Fainsinger RL and Kastelan C (1992) Palliative care rounds: custom-made suppositories of methadone for severe cancer pain. *Journal of Pain and Symptom Management* **7**(6): 372–4.

15 Edwards JC and Marier RL (ed.) (1989) *Clinical teaching for medical residents roles, techniques and programs*. New York: Springer Publishing Co.

16 Fainsinger R, Chan K and Bruera E (1992) Total parenteral nutrition for a terminally ill patient. *Journal of Palliative Care* **8**(2): 30–2.

17 Weinholtz D and Edwards JC (1992) *Teaching during rounds*. A handbook for attending physicians and residents. Baltimore: The Johns Hopkins University Press.

18 MacEachern E (1992) *A study to determine the reliability and validity of the Edmonton Symptom Assessment System (ESAS)*. Abstract. Presented at the 9th International Congress on care of the terminally ill, Montreal, Canada, October 31–November 4.

9

Audit Methods: Palliative Care Core Standards

JOHN HUNT*

Introduction

This chapter will describe the formation of the Trent Hospice Audit Group, its decision to write core standards for palliative care and the development of the standards and audit tools to publication as 'Palliative care core standards – a multidisciplinary approach'. Two of the six standards are included in full.

The chapter includes examples of the difficulties that the group encountered during the evolution of the standards writing and in initial attempts to introduce a 'top-down' development into individual hospices within the Trent Region. It concludes with a description of the way in which our group intends to take the work forward and the initial steps taken in the auditing process.

*On behalf of Trent Hospice Audit Group

Dr Robert Catterall, St Barnabas' Hospice
Mrs Jean Freeman, Ashgate Hospice
Mrs Margaret Carradice, St Luke's Hospice
Mrs Bronwyn Biswas, Leicestershire Hospice
Dr Tony Crowther, St Luke's Hospice
Mrs Margaret Duffy, Staunton Harold Hospice
Dr G Rathbone, Staunton Harold Hospice

Dr Joanna Hocknall, Nottingham Hospice
Dr Vaughan Keeley, Macmillan Continuing Care Unit
Mrs Penny McFaul, St Barnabas' Hospice
Dr Sam Ahmedzai, Leicestershire Hospice
Dr Richard Atkinson, Ashgate Hospice

The Trent Hospice Audit Group

The Trent Hospice Audit Group (THAG) came together after two groups – one of consultants in palliative medicine/medical directors, the other of matrons/senior nurses – from regional hospices had attempted as single disciplines to work on audit measures for medical/clinical issues. Both groups quickly realized that Ford's statement 'as palliative care is a multiprofessional activity, it has been accepted that audit must, therefore, be multiprofessional also'[1], was correct and the THAG was formed in late 1990. It was agreed that it should have regular monthly meetings in a central unit within the region.

Recognizing the importance of audit, and particularly, the need to make explicit statements relating to quality of service and the service values in the (at that time) newly developing purchaser/provider relationships within health authorities, the group's initial focus was on two pieces of work, 'documentation standards' (see Chapter 7) and 'palliative care core standards'.

Why core standards?

The group chose to write core standards for several reasons:

- we wanted to identify the basic, most important parts of our philosophy, service and values
- we wanted to have realistic numbers of standards to set, and attempt to achieve
- our hope was that all hospices within the Trent Region would take ownership of the completed core standards, and develop clinical standards within their own teams depending upon local needs, bearing in mind that standards should be agreed or set by those to whom they will apply. Standards can only be achieved and improved upon if there is commitment to them from those responsible for their implementation
- we wanted, ultimately, to obtain the best possible service for the groups of patients that use it, and effect an improvement in the quality of care
- THAG felt able to attempt to develop these core standards given our clear and shared understanding of the goals, purposes and values of our organization, the hospice, and our sound knowledge of the specialty

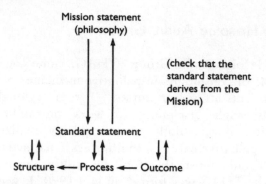

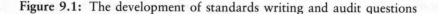

Figure 9.1: The development of standards writing and audit questions

- in embarking on our core standards writing we adopted Dona-bedian's model of *Structure – Process – Outcome*. Figure 9.1 demonstrates how we attempted to develop our standard and criteria statements, and at the same time, fashion our audit tool questions. By attempting to use this model as a way of checking back to ensure that criteria statements related to the standard statement and that, similarly, the standard statement related to the mission (philosophy) statement, we hoped to avoid errors and confusion, and to give clarity to the work.

The Palliative Care Core Standards

Whilst each of the six Trent hospices involved in writing the standards had very individual mission statements, all reflected the *core* parts of the philosophy of palliative care. Therefore, deciding on six standards to develop was not a difficult process. Box 9.1 gives the six standard statement headings. Standard statements 1 to 5 are related directly to palliative care patients and carers, while statement 6 is an organizational standard.

Box 9.1: Palliative Care Core Standards

Standard statement headings:

1. Collaboration with other agencies.
2. Symptom control.
3. Patient/carer information.
4. Emotional support.
5. Bereavement care and support.
6. Specialist education for staff.

Before offering examples of the standards and their audit tools, it would seem appropriate to mention some of the difficulties encountered by the group in relation to the practicalities of the work development and timescale.

The THAG had difficulty in moving through the standard writing stages and so the timescale for completing six standards was long, approximately 15 months. The major hurdles were:

- choosing a sub-group to work on drafts of the statements and criteria
- maintaining an awareness of the need to take care with language (say what you mean, mean what you say) and tense, in fashioning the statements. The importance of having a dictionary to hand when writing standards cannot be emphasized enough
- knowing when to take work back to the larger group for discussion. Our experience suggests that the sub-groups should not labour too long on the draft work if the cohesion of the group as a whole is to be maintained
- having a clear working procedure for the sections (criteria) and the whole standard in relation to the principles of standard writing (*see* Figure 9.1). This enabled the group to refine as necessary, but also to know when to stop
- recognizing that the standards which the group completed were a 'starting point' and that the progression of the audit cycle would lead over time to a greater revision and refinement of the tools.

From the six palliative care core standards, two examples are now shown, Standards No. 2 symptom control (*see* Box 9.2) and No. 4 emotional support (*see* Box 9.3). Appendix H shows the Palliative Care Core Standards statements.

Box 9.2: Standard No. 2 – symptom control

Care group: Palliative care patients

Standard statement: All patients have their symptoms controlled to a degree that is acceptable to them, and achievable by multidisciplinary team intervention within current palliative care knowledge.

Criteria:

Structure   A suitably qualified team member, known and acceptable to the patient, is readily available for advice on symptom management.

The team member has undertaken post-registration training, and is competent in symptom control.

The team member has enhanced communication skills.

Process   The multidisciplinary team assesses the patient symptoms. Together with the patient, or his advocate, the team formulates and documents a plan of care.

The team monitors and reviews the care plan and liaises with other health care professionals as necessary.

Outcome   The patient, or his advocate, states that his symptoms are controlled to a level acceptable to him/them (from List 1).

There is evidence that a multidisciplinary team approach, involving the patient and/or his advocate, was used.

Audit: Outcome audit:

1. The patient, or his advocate, state that the symptoms are controlled to a level acceptable to him/them (from List 1).   Yes/No

   Audit question – 'Has your . . . been controlled?'

2. There is evidence that a multidisciplinary team approach, involving the patient, and/or his advocate, was used.

   Audit from documentation.

Process audit:

1. Is there evidence that the patient's care plan was reviewed or revised by the multidisciplinary team?
                                                              Yes/No

   Audit from documentation.

2. Is there evidence that the patient, or his advocate, was involved in formulating a plan of care?
                                                              Yes/No

---

Box 9.2: *continued*

> Audit question − 'Did the (doctor/nurse) explain what we were able to do, and ask what you wanted us to do?'
3. Did the team document a plan of care?   Yes/No
   Audit from documentation.
4. Is there evidence that a multidisciplinary team approach was used to assess the patient's symptoms?
   Yes/No

> Audit − from documentation.
> Question for team members − 'Are there multidisciplinary meetings?'

Box 9.3: Standard No. 4 − emotional support

Care group:	Palliative care patients and carers
Standard statement:	The patient and his carers have access, to expertise in counselling, psychological and spiritual care, to provide emotional support.
Criteria:	
Structure	Within the multidisciplinary team, there are members with specialized counselling and communication skills.
	A room, or area, is designed to allow privacy for the patient and key worker.
	Sufficient time is negotiated and made available.
Process	The multidisciplinary team assess and prioritize emotional support needs with the patient and carer/s.
	The team nominates a key worker/s, dependent on the expertise required.
	The supportive aspects of care are documented in the care plan by both the nursing and key worker team members, and there is evidence of multidisciplinary evaluation.
	Referral to other specialist professionals as indicated eg psychiatrists or psychologists, is negotiated with the patient or carer and arranged by the key worker.

Box 9.3: *continued*

	There is liaison and feedback from specialist interaction with the patient or carer.
	Team and key members ensure that confidentiality is maintained within the team.
Outcome	The patient states that he had the opportunity to raise emotional difficulties.
	The patient has access to support from a key worker with expertise related to the emotional need.
	The carer states that he has had the opportunity to raise emotional difficulties.
	Yes/No
	The carer has access to support from a key worker with expertise related to the emotional need.
	The patient or carer is aware that confidentiality is maintained within the team, or key members.
	The key worker states that there has been some relief or resolution of psychosocial issues.
Audit:	Outcome audit:
	1. The patient states that he has had the opportunity to raise emotional difficulties.
	Yes/No
	Audit question – 'Have you been able to raise any difficult emotional issues?
	Outcome audit (continued):
	2. The patient has access to support from a key worker with expertise related to the emotional need.
	Yes/No
	Audit from documentation.
	3. The carer states that he has had the opportunity to raise emotional difficulties.
	Yes/No
	Audit question – as for outcome.
	4. The carer has access to support from a key worker with expertise related to the emotional need. Yes/No

Box 9.3: *continued*

Audit from documentation.

5. The patient, or carer, is aware that confidentiality is maintained within the team, or key members.

Yes/No

Audit question to patient.

6. The key worker states that there has been some relief or resolution of psychosocial issues.

Yes/No

Audit from documentation.

Process audit:

1. Is there evidence of a multidisciplinary team assessment of the emotional support needs of the patient and his/her carer/s?

Yes/No

Audit from documentation.

2. Was prioritization of the emotional needs negotiated with the patient, and/or his/her carer/s?

Yes/No

3. Were key workers identified from within the team, dependent upon the need?

Yes/No

Audit from documentation.

4. Was there documentation of sessions with the patient or carer/s?

Yes/No

Audit from documentation.

5. Was there negotiation and agreement about the role of external specialist professionals with the patient and carer/s before referral?

Yes/No

Audit from documentation.

Specialist agencies were able to accept the referral, to report and liaise. The patient and/or carer state that they were helped by the agencies involved. Multidisciplinary team review confirms the specialist agencies' effectiveness.

What next?

Having published the standards document as a starting point, the THAG was fortunate in being able to secure funding for two posts which will enable us to develop, implement, test and validate the work.

In association with the Trent Palliative Care Centre, an audit officer post (funded by Help the Hospices for a two-year period) will enable research into the best methods of implementing audit within the Trent hospices and will give us the opportunity to learn from, and adopt, good practice in audit measures from sources outside our region. The initial part of this project involves the officer conducting semi-structured interviews with nurses and other multidisciplinary team members, to establish a baseline awareness of audit. The postholder will also make a major contribution to the revision and refinement of the standard statements and criteria.

In addition, the group has secured the services of an audit facilitator (funded from regional medical audit monies) which will enable standardized auditing in each of the group's hospices (we have grown to eight in-patient units) at regular intervals.

A steering group, with the facilitator and officer, are developing the auditing process along two lines – those questions related to the standards statement and criteria which can be audited from documentation (medical, nursing notes, etc), and developing an interview structure for patients/carers using the suggested wording from the audit tools. Finally, for anyone interested in following the THAG's example of writing standards, take care in the introduction of the work into a unit. Whilst our group had commitment to, and ownership of the work, our 'top-down' approach meant that care and time was needed in offering the standards to individual hospice teams.

A variety of presentation methods have been used including combining an introduction to the standards document with a review of a hospice mission statement and introducing a single standard at team meetings. This long period of familiarization has caused some frustration but is vital if audit is to become meaningful to our speciality.

References

1 Ford G (1990) Constructive audit. *Palliative Medicine* 4(1): Editorial.

Further reading

'*Palliative Care Core Standards – a multidisciplinary approach*', The Trent Hospice Audit Group. See below for supply address.

For additional information contact the author – Nightingale Macmillan Continuing Care Unit, 117A London Road, Derby DE1 2QS. Telephone: Derby (0332) 254911.

10

Audit Methods: Views of the Family after the Death

JULIA ADDINGTON-HALL AND MARK McCARTHY

Introduction

It is increasingly recognized within the NHS that it is important to know what the consumers of services – patients themselves – think about the services provided. In palliative care, particular emphasis is put on the importance of seeing patients and their families as partners in the care process who, wherever possible, should be enabled to make choices about the care they receive. It is, therefore, especially appropriate that the views of patients and their families should be sought when collecting information on the quality and appropriateness of palliative care.

Whose views to collect – those of patients or families?

Asking patients for their views of the services they receive in the last days and weeks of life is not without difficulties. These are summarized in Box 10.1. Although there are several examples of studies which have successfully sought the views of dying people[1,2] it is often more feasible to collect information from relatives. Interviewing relatives before the patient's death can, however, present some of the same problems as those found when interviewing the patients themselves – it can be difficult to get a representative sample, it may seem intrusive, and relatives may be reluctant to criticize doctors and nurses on whom the patient's comfort depends. An alternative approach which overcomes many of these problems is to talk to relatives after the death of the patient. This has the advantage that a representative sample of deaths in a particular palliative care unit or health district can be included and information can be collected on the whole period leading up to the death. This approach is not without its drawbacks as outlined in Box 10.2. However, as shown by the examples given below, it is feasible to interview bereaved relatives about the quality of care provided in a district or by a palliative care service, and the information collected in this way can play an important role in auditing palliative care.

Box 10.1: Difficulties in using patients to collect information on the quality of palliative care services

1. It can be intrusive to ask patients in their last weeks of life to complete a questionnaire or to be interviewed.
2. Many are too ill to participate by the time they are receiving palliative care services. For instance, 35% of a group of cancer patients with a life expectancy of less than a year died before they could be interviewed[3]. This means that any survey of patients is likely to be unrepresentative – it will include only those patients well enough to take part.
3. It can be difficult to ask patients who do not know or acknowledge their diagnosis or prognosis about their experience of palliative care without raising concerns that this will inappropriately alert them to the nature of their illness. Again, this means that patients included in a survey of palliative care are likely to be unrepresentative of all patients receiving these services.
4. Patients may be reluctant to criticize their care, despite reassurances of confidentiality. They may be concerned that their care may be adversely affected if staff get to hear of their criticisms, or may feel that any complaints are a sign of ingratitude.

Box 10.2: Limitations in using bereaved relatives as a source of information on palliative care services

1. There are dangers in treating relatives' views as if they accurately represent those of the patients themselves. Even before bereavement relatives' views of symptom control and service satisfaction are likely to differ from patients' views. For instance, patients have been found to give pain significantly lower ratings than their relatives[4]. Little is known about how and in what ways relatives' and patients' views diverge and how this is affected by bereavement.

Box 10.2: *Continued*

2. Bereaved relatives' views of care will be influenced by bereavement and may differ from their own views before the patient's death. Negative memories come to mind more readily at times of sadness and this may lead to relatives putting more weight on times when things went wrong than on times when care was good. Little is known about the effects of bereavement on how care before the patient's death is remembered and judged. Equally, little is known about how this is influenced by time from death, although the number and extent of differences have been shown to be small in responses to questions on symptoms, need for help and care received, between interviews conducted three and nine months after the death[5].

3. Some people feel that bereaved people will be distressed by being reminded of the death, and that consequently it is not ethical to ask their views of patient care. However, experience from several large studies which have interviewed bereaved people suggests that the vast majority appreciate the opportunity to talk about the deceased[6].

Examples of successful surveys of bereaved relatives

There are several examples of interview surveys of bereaved relatives which have shed light on local service provision. For example, 80 bereaved relatives of cancer patients were interviewed in a study carried out in one large district general hospital and results showed that symptom control was a major problem, that the existing community services were inadequate to enable all patients to be at home when desired, and that improvements were needed in the care of dying patients on acute wards[7]. In another study, 37 lay carers of patients in a hospice were interviewed after bereavement[8]. Although most lay carers were satisfied, they were less satisfied with care from community nurses and GPs than from hospice staff, and a minority had had little contact with hospice staff and were dissatisfied with information they had received. Criticisms about communication with professionals were also reported in an interview survey of 106 bereaved relatives of people dying in one health district, as were inadequate symptom control and a lack of bereavement support[9]. Each of these surveys has played an important role in auditing local services by identifying areas where services were failing to meet the needs of patients and relatives.

Interview surveys versus postal questionnaires

Surveys which collect the views of up to 200 people are within the capability of palliative care services, given sufficient planning and adequate resources. The latter will, however, often be a constraint. Because of the need to employ interviewers and to cover their travelling expenses, which may be considerable for palliative care services with large catchment areas, interview surveys are costly. They also require considerable resources and expertise for data entry and processing, analysis and interpretation. An alternative is to use self-completion questionnaires which can be mailed to bereaved relatives.

These are considerably cheaper than interviews, need fewer trained staff to administer and analyse, and remove any danger of interviewer bias. However, postal questionnaires have a number of disadvantages – there is no opportunity for clarification of ambiguities in answers or for exploring the reasons respondents hold the views they do. There is also no guarantee that the questionnaire will be completed by the most appropriate person and no way of checking this. For these reasons it has been claimed that an interview will always be better than a self-complete questionnaire in obtaining sensitive information accurately. However, Fitzpatrick has argued that there is no reason why a carefully developed self-completion questionnaire should be as second best as this suggests[10]. There is little experience so far in using postal questionnaires with bereaved people and it is not clear that they would find completing a questionnaire acceptable – they may prefer a face-to-face interview in which they have the opportunity to discuss their concerns and to talk about the deceased[4]. Questionnaires which are seen as invasive or insensitive are unlikely to be returned. It is more difficult to follow-up non-responders in a postal survey – interviewers may be able to track down someone if, as is common after bereavement, they have moved but there is no way of doing this with a postal survey. Response rates may therefore be lower than in an interview survey. The question of whether to conduct a postal or interview survey has no straightforward answer and will depend largely upon the resources available.

Questions to consider before starting a survey of bereaved relatives

Regardless of which approach is taken a number of questions need to be considered before beginning such a study. These are outlined in Box 10.3. It is easy to underestimate the time needed to locate and interview people or to send out questionnaires and reminders, the resources needed to analyse the information collected, and the skills needed to interpret the results. Remember that useful information can be obtained from a small exploratory survey, as long as those included are representative of the relatives of patients using the service. Consider also whether a quantitative survey involving numbers and data analysis is really needed – could the service's requirements be met by a descriptive study in which the views of relatives are collated and described but not coded for statistical analysis?

It is important not to undertake a survey of relatives without considering carefully the aims of the survey, the resources available and

---

Box 10.3: Points to consider before embarking on a survey of bereaved relatives

1. How can relatives be selected so that they are representative of relatives of patients using the service?
2. What are the aims of the exercise? What aspects of the service is it concerned with? Which of these are essential to cover and which could be left out if the questionnaire or interview schedule becomes too long?
3. Is it possible to use existing questionnaires such as that used in the Regional Study of Care for the Dying (RSCD), or questions from them? If new questions are needed, have books on questionnaire design been consulted and/or expert advice sought? Have the questions been piloted to ensure they are acceptable, mean what the investigator thinks, and cover issues the respondents think are important? Have the reliability and validity of the questions been considered?
4. Do additional items of information such as the relationship of the deceased to the relative need to be collected to help in the interpretation of the results?
5. How is the information going to be handled once it is collected? Will it be coded and entered on a computer? If so, how and by whom? What computer software will be used?
6. How will the information be analysed? Are statistics going to be used and, if so, which? Is advice on this needed?
7. Has adequate time been allowed? Are there adequate resources, both in terms of money and people?
8. Is ethical committee approval needed? Should local GPs be informed? Does the study need to be registered under the Data Protection Act?
9. How will the results of the survey be fed back to the palliative care service? What is the mechanism for ensuring that action is taken, if necessary?

what advice is needed and from whom it can be gained. There are a number of good references on survey design and questionnaire development, some of which are listed below. It is recommended that some of these are consulted at the planning stage of the study in order to help prevent the investigator from drowning under an over-ambitious project or designing one which produces misleading results.

What action will result from the survey?

One of the risks of asking relatives for their views of palliative care services is that they will not always give the answers the staff expected or ones which the staff find easy to accept. At times, this may lead to a temptation to ignore the results or to find reasons why the answers are biased or misleading. Again, this makes it important for the study to be designed and executed in a way that minimizes bias and maximizes the amount of confidence that can be placed in its findings. Another common temptation is to argue that the problems have been dealt with in the time that has elapsed between the relatives being consulted and the results becoming available and that consequently the results are now irrelevant. Surveys do indeed get out of date and it is important to feed results back as quickly as possible, both to avoid them becoming outdated and to avoid others using this as an argument for ignoring results they do not like. There is no point asking relatives for their views of services unless these will be listened to, and this means that the ways in which their views will be fed back to the service providers and the mechanisms for acting upon the results should be considered before beginning a survey.

The remainder of this chapter will use the example of the Regional Study of Care for the Dying (RSCD), the largest interview survey of bereaved relatives to date in the United Kingdom, to illustrate some of the stages involved in an interview survey, to demonstrate the feasibility of interviewing relatives and to show how information collected in this way can play an important role in auditing palliative care.

The Regional Study of Care for the Dying

Aims

This study was set up at University College London in 1990 primarily to provide health districts with information to enable them to compare their provision for the dying with that provided by other districts. Other aims included the development of outcome measures for death and bereavement which could be used routinely by districts and service providers for quality assurance; the description of the needs of people dying from conditions other than cancer; and the evaluation of the effectiveness of specialist palliative care services. District health authorities (DHAs) in England were invited to take part in the study on the basis that in return for a participation fee the services they provided for the dying would be audited. Twenty districts chose to join the study.

Methods

The methods used in the study built upon those used in two studies by Ann Cartwright who interviewed surviving relatives of a nationally representative sample of deaths in 1969 to describe the last year of life and the adequacy of service provision[3], and repeated the study in 1987 to see what changes had happened in the intervening years[4]. It was decided to use the same methods and essentially the same interview schedule in the RSCD because these had been shown to be effective, to be capable of detecting change over time[11] and therefore likely to be able to detect differences between districts, and to provide a wealth of valuable information. It would also be possible to compare district results with those of the nationally representative 1987 data.

Ethical committees

Both the RSCD and the 1987 survey started rather later than anticipated because of delays in obtaining ethical committee approval in participating districts. While some committees were satisfied that the studies presented no major ethical problems and that the proposed study design took adequate account of both the need to be sensitive to bereaved relatives and the need to ensure informed consent was obtained, others expressed considerable alarm at the idea of intruding on the grief of bereaved people. Although permission was finally obtained in all the RSCD districts, two ethical committees approached in the 1987 survey refused permission for the study to go ahead in their areas[4]. Although it is understandable and indeed appropriate that concerns should be expressed about intruding on people's grief, the experience of both studies is that the vast majority of respondents found the opportunity to talk to a sympathetic interviewer about the deceased useful.

Clearly, in such a sensitive area careful consideration needs to be given to ethical considerations. This will include the issue of how best to approach people – in the RSCD a letter was sent to the deceased's address before the interviewer called; whilst in the 1987 survey the interviewer called without prior warning. The letter enabled people who did not want to take part to telephone the research team immediately, but it also left some relatives concerned about the study or upset by being reminded of their loss without any immediate opportunity to discuss their anxieties with an interviewer. In addition, the letter undoubtedly contributed to the fall in response rate from 80% in 1987 to 69%. Although the reduced response rate may be seen as appropriate – relatives may have felt less able to refuse when approached by an interviewer and therefore were in more danger of feeling coerced to take part – a fall in response rate also has ethical implications: the scientific validity of a study is reduced as the response rate falls and it is unethical to ask people to take part in a study which is of limited validity because of its response rate. Surveys of bereaved relatives do raise difficult ethical issues but, in contrast to the opinion expressed by some ethical committees, the vast majority of respondents seem to find the interview a positive rather than entirely negative experience.

The sample

Within each district, 270 deaths were sampled randomly from the death certificates of residents aged 16 or over who died in the last quarter of 1990, giving a total sample size of 5378. As cancer patients are the focus of most palliative care services more cancer deaths than non-cancer deaths were sampled. Between seven and 13 months after the death, the DHA sent a letter to the address of the deceased to introduce the study and trained interviewers then contacted the address to find the person who knew most about the deceased's last 12 months of life and, if they were willing, to interview them. They succeeded in interviewing someone in 69% of the sample, and they reported that for 89% of these the person they interviewed had been the most appropriate person to tell them about the last year of life. Wives or husbands were interviewed about 36% of the deceased, children about 30%, other relatives about 16%, friends or neighbours about 9%, and officials about the remaining 10%.

The interview schedule

As deaths were sampled randomly from death certificates, they included the full range of adult deaths from the sudden death of a young person in a motorbike accident to the expected death of an elderly person who had lived in a nursing home for years, had complex medical problems and repeated hospital admissions. Consequently the interview schedule, adapted for use from that used by Cartwright and Seale[4] needed to include a wide selection of questions, most of which were relevant only to a sub-section of the sample (*see* Box 10.4 for topics covered in the schedule). The complexity of the schedule, together with the need to be sensitive to the concerns of the bereaved relatives, meant that the survey needed particularly skilful interviewers. Most of the interview schedule

---

Box 10.4: The Regional Study of Care for the Dying interview schedule

A *Contents of the interview schedule*

- sources of formal and informal care, and respondents' experience of caring for the person who died
- symptoms and symptom control
- restrictions experienced by the person who died, and the help they received with these
- experience of, and satisfaction with, community nursing services, in-patient hospital and hospice care, out-patient, day centre and GP care
- information from, and communication with, health professionals
- relatives' experiences of bereavement and bereavement care.

B *Example of question included in interview schedule*

'Altogether, and taking all things into consideration, would you say the care Mrs Jones received, in the year before she died, from the health and social services was:

excellent	1
good	2
fair	3
poor	4
(other	5)

---

was structured and, in order to minimize bias arising from the way questions were asked, interviewers were instructed to ask questions exactly as written and in the order they were written. The respondent was asked to choose the most appropriate answer from a number of options given and the interviewer then circled the corresponding number on the schedule, thus reducing the coding needed before responses could be entered on a computer for analysis. A number of open questions were included to help ensure that the respondent had the opportunity to mention issues not otherwise covered, and interviewers were encouraged to record responses to these questions verbatim. Such questions take time and resources to code but can give reports arising from the survey a more 'human' feel, as well as highlighting issues omitted from the schedule because they were not on the investigators' agenda.

Once the schedules were returned to the research team, they were checked for errors and omissions, coded where necessary and entered on a database. These computer files were also carefully checked for errors before data analysis, using the statistical package SPSS-PC, began.

Considerable research, interviewing and computer expertise are required by a study of this size and complexity. However, as already discussed, useful results can also come out of much smaller surveys.

Feedback to districts

The districts who took part in the RSCD did so because they wanted information on how need for, and satisfaction with, their services for the dying compared with that elsewhere. Providing them with feedback was, therefore, one of the main aims of the study. Each district received a comprehensive package of feedback which compared the district's score on each question to that for the study as a whole, for cancer and non-cancer deaths separately. In order to help districts interpret their results the feedback was accompanied by a description of service provision in each district and an explanation of how response bias may have affected the results.

Results from one of the first districts to receive their feedback, District 'A', will now be considered, showing the value of including the views of relatives in an audit of local services for the dying.

Using data from the RSCD to audit local services

District A is in an urban area with high levels of unemployment and deprivation. A smaller proportion of spouses were interviewed than in the study as a whole which may have led to the district seeming to do less than was actually the case. Study data show that spouses are less critical of services than other relatives or friends. There were, however, no differences in response bias between this district and all districts combined, so there are no other reasons to doubt the validity of comparisons between the district's data and that for all the districts combined.

Six problem areas were identified where scores in District A were significantly lower than in the study as a whole. These are listed in Box 10.5, together with the main ways in which the characteristics of the sample in this district differed from the total study sample. Some of the problem areas are undoubtedly a consequence of these differences – for instance, a high unmet need for help with selfcare and domestic tasks was probably due at least in part to a large number of people living alone and a high incidence of dementia.

When these results were fed back to the district they confirmed some local suspicions about, for example, the need for more social service support and some GPs providing a worse service than was desirable. The district was pleased to have 'hard' numerical evidence to support what had been previously only hunches about problem areas. However, the results also highlighted areas which previously had not been of concern, such as the failure to give adequate and clear information to

Box 10.5: Using the Regional Study of Care for the Dying data to audit care for the dying provided by District 'A'

Areas of concern identified from comparisons of District A's data with that for all districts combined

1. High levels of unmet need for help with activities of selfcare (such as washing and dressing) and domestic tasks – despite average service provision and above average involvement from relatives.
2. High dissatisfaction with the service provided by GPs – especially as regards their willingness to visit and a lack of understanding of the patient's problems.
3. Poor symptom control – both in hospital and in the community.
4. Lack of information to relatives.
5. Lack of choice about treatment and place of death.
6. High self-perceived burden on informal carers.

Ways in which the sample in this district differed from the total sample

1. High numbers of hospice deaths and low numbers of deaths in residential and nursing homes.
2. Few deaths of people over 85 from cancer, and more lung cancer deaths.
3. Lower social class.
4. More people who died from cancer lived alone.
5. More support from relatives living outside the household.
6. More people suffered from confusion in the last year of life, and dementia was mentioned on more death certificates.
7. More people were resident in hospital for a year or more, and fewer were resident in a residential or nursing home for the same period.
8. Lower overall quality of life in the last year of life.

relatives, and a perceived lack of choice for either patients or families about the type of treatments received and the place of death. Following the presentation of these data, both purchasers and providers began to consider ways in which these problem areas could be tackled. A similar survey in the future would close the 'audit cycle' (*see* Chapter 2) and show the extent to which it has been possible to produce improvements at a time of financial constraint.

Conclusion

This chapter has considered the advantages of including the views of relatives in audits of palliative care and has drawn on the experience of the RSCD to show that doing so is not only feasible but can also generate useful results about local services. Whilst a large survey will be outside the capabilities of most palliative care services many will be able to undertake small interview or postal surveys of bereaved relatives of patients who have received their services, given sufficient planning and resources. Relatives give a valuable perspective on palliative care services and their views can help prevent professionals falling into the trap of providing the services they think are required, rather than those which actually are. The difficulties of collecting the views of relatives in a systematic way can seem overwhelming, but the benefits of doing so can greatly outweigh the problems on route.

References

1 Higginson I, Wade A and McCarthy M (1990) Palliative care: views of patients and their families. *British Medical Journal* 301: 277–80.

2 Townsend J, Frank AO, Fermont D, Dyer S, Karan O, Walgrove A and Piper M (1990) Terminal cancer care and patients' preference for place of death: a prospective study. *British Medical Journal* 301: 415–17.

3 Addington-Hall JM, MacDonald LD, Anderson HR, Chamberlain J, Freeling P, Bland JM and Raftery J (1992) Randomised controlled trial of effects of co-ordinating care for terminally ill cancer patients. *British Medical Journal* 305: 1317–21.

4 Curtis AE and Fernster J (1989) Quality of life of oncology hospice patients: a comparison of patient and primary caregiver reports. *Oncol Nurs Forum* 16: '49–53.

5 Cartwright A, Hockey L and Anderson JL (1973) *Life before death*. London: Routledge and Kegan Paul.

6 Cartwright A and Seale C (1990) *The natural history of a survey*. London: King's Fund Centre.

7 Addington-Hall JM, MacDonald LD, Anderson HR and Freeling P (1991) Dying from cancer: the views of bereaved family and friends about the experience of terminally ill patients. *Palliative Medicine* 5: 207–14.

8 Field D, Dand P, Ahmedzai S and Biswas B (1992) Care and information received by lay carers of terminally ill patients at the Leicestershire hospice. *Palliative Medicine* 6: 237–45.

9 Sykes NP, Pearson SE and Chell S (1992) Quality of care of the terminally ill: the carer's perspective. *Palliative Medicine* 6: 227–36.

10 Fitzpatrick R (1991) Surveys of patient satisfaction: I – Important general considerations. *British Medical Journal* 302: 887–9.

11 Cartwright A (1991) Changes in life and care in the year before death 1969–1987. *Journal of Public Health Medicine* 13: 81–7.

Further reading

Abramson JH (1990) *Survey methods in community medicine* (4th edition). London: Churchill Livingstone.

Fitzpatrick R (1991) Surveys of patient satisfaction: II – Designing a questionnaire and conducting a survey. *British Medical Journal* 302: 1129–32.

Moser C and Kalton G (1971) *Survey methods in social investigation*. Aldershot: Gower Publishing Group.

St Leger AS, Schnieden H and Walsworth-Bell JP (1992) *Evaluating health services' effectiveness*. Milton Keynes: Open University Press.

11

Audit Methods: HIV/AIDS Care

ELIZABETH BUTTERS, ROBERT GEORGE AND IRENE HIGGINSON

This chapter describes how an existing validated audit measure, the Support Team Assessment Schedule (STAS) (*see* Chapter 5), was adapted for use with teams providing care to HIV/AIDS patients. Findings from an evaluation of two HIV/AIDS teams are presented to demonstrate the use of the resulting audit.

Introduction

In the late 1980s two central London health districts (Bloomsbury and Parkside) established community support teams for people with HIV/AIDS. The Bloomsbury Community Care Team (CCT) and St Mary's Home Support Team (HST) were the first teams of their kind (*see* Box 11.1). Both teams took part in an evaluation which aimed to describe and compare their working arrangements and the characteristics of patients referred, and to provide information on the needs of HIV/AIDS patients and the effectiveness of services.

Why adapt an existing measure?

Adapting an existing validated measure has several advantages: it saves time, so that audit can begin more quickly and allows for comparison with any existing data.

The STAS was originally developed with and used by the Bloomsbury cancer home support team (*see* Chapter 5) and Bloomsbury Health Authority were keen for the new HIV/AIDS team (CCT) to be evaluated in a similar way.

Box 11.1: HIV/AIDS teams

Two multidisciplinary teams in central London developed following palliative care and hospice models to assist in the care of people with HIV/AIDS.

Community Care Team (CCT)

- community unit base
- originally consisted of a consultant, two clinical nurse specialists, a social worker (the social worker post was later replaced by an additional nursing position), an administrator and a research assistant
- a dietitian, occupational therapist and registrar later joined the CCT.

Home Support Team (HST)

- original base: HIV/AIDS clinic. Later moved to a hospital base
- originally consisted of a senior nurse co-ordinator, five nursing sisters or charge nurses, a part-time clinical assistant (with other hospital duties), and administrative support
- a part-time welfare rights worker and occupational therapist later joined HST.

Both teams accept referrals from hospital and community staff and care for patients both at home and when they are in hospital. They provide specialist advice and support, working with other professionals rather than taking over their clinical responsibilities.

The STAS was adapted, rather than a new measure developed so that:

- evaluation could begin more quickly (ie the audit would be part of the team's working practice from the beginning)
- the STAS could be revalidated with HIV/AIDS patients
- data from HIV/AIDS and cancer teams could be compared to consider the different problems and needs of cancer and HIV/AIDS patients.

Adapting the measure

When adapting an existing measure a number of factors must be taken into consideration:

- patient and carer characteristics
- nature of the illness/disease under consideration
- working practice (ie composition and role)
- relevance of audit items and their definitions
- frequency of assessments
- reliability and validity.

Initially we worked with the Bloomsbury CCT to:

- identify the main differences between cancer and HIV/AIDS patients
- consider the working practices of the HIV/AIDS team and how the STAS could be incorporated into them
- consider the relevance of STAS items and their definitions of HIV/AIDS patients and teams
- identify and try to resolve any problems which HIV/AIDS teams might face whilst using the STAS to audit their work.

An independent researcher (EB) observed the team's working practice, including their weekly patient discussion meeting, for a number of weeks. Discussions were held with individual team members and the team as a whole, to determine how the STAS should be adapted and how best to incorporate the audit into their working practice.

The characteristics of HIV/AIDS patients and their carers, along with the nature of HIV infection and its treatment lead to a number of problems when assessing some STAS items. Box 11.2 shows some of the main differences between cancer and HIV/AIDS patients.

STAS items which were modified

The following STAS items required modification (or presented problems in the way in which they were assessed):

- family anxiety
- family insight
- patient anxiety
- patient insight
- communication between patient and family
- communication from professionals to patient and family
- planning
- predictability
- spiritual.

Box 11.2: Main differences between HIV/AIDS and cancer patients

HIV/AIDS patients tend to:

- be younger (mean age 37.5 years HIV/AIDS, 66 years cancer)[1]
- have more complicated networks of carers (ie carers are often partners, friends or parents, who may be in conflict with each other) and social problems (eg isolation, stigma, loss of employment and income, financial and housing problems, multiple losses etc)
- spend longer in care (mean time 16 CCT/41 HST weeks HIV/AIDS, 7 weeks cancer)[1]
- have a wider variety of medical presentations and problems (common symptoms include: weakness, diarrhoea, muscle wasting, depression/anxiety, memory loss, visual problems and dyspnoea)[1] (*see* also Figures 11.1 and 11.2)
- require more complicated management. Patients are frequently prescribed five to ten different drugs per day as part of acute therapy, maintenance or prophylaxis. Sophisticated drug regimes may change rapidly and use of long-term prophylaxis is common[2]. Use of intravenous therapy, Hickman lines, total parenteral nutrition and blood transfusions is also common
- be difficult to prognosticate for (and to identify the terminal phase)
- have a lower degree of GP (family doctor) involvement.

Teams may experience some difficulty in deciding for whom STAS family items (ie anxiety and insight) should be assessed for. HIV/AIDS patients' lay or informal carers are often different from those associated with cancer patients. The majority of HIV/AIDS patients are cared for by partners, parents or friends. Patients may have complex networks of carers and their main carer may change over time. Family items are assessed for the principle carer at the time of assessment and teams note who this is. To allow teams to record situations where a number of carers are involved the teams note the presence of any significant others, in addition to the nearest carer.

Minor alterations were made to the definitions for communication between patient and family, to include situations where patients were communicating with their partners openly, but not as openly, or if at all, with their family members.

Patient insight, patient anxiety, communication between patient and family and communication from professionals to patient and family may become difficult or impossible to assess when patients are suffering from dementia, confusion or short-term memory loss (common symptoms of some HIV opportunistic infections). In these circumstances the items are recorded as missing and teams note the onset of dementia.

Sometimes when patients are suffering from dementia it may be necessary to assess planning and predictability from the team's point of view, rather than the patient's, to record urgent needs and problems which the patient may be unaware of.

Predictability, planning, patient insight and family insight may be particularly difficult to assess if the team do not know when a patient is likely to die. Teams find it very difficult to prognosticate (ie give a prognosis range) for HIV/AIDS patients. Patients can suffer from periods of acute illness when they seem close to death, indeed to dying, and then make a sudden recovery. Some patients can have a very sudden and rapid terminal phase. We found that unlike cancer teams, HIV/AIDS teams did not try to give a prognosis range for their patients. They found it very difficult to assess predictability and this item has subsequently been removed from the STAS.

One item, spiritual, only had provisional definitions, and was not widely assessed by cancer teams (see Chapter 5). The HIV/AIDS team were keen to improve the definitions for this item as they felt that it was an important aspect of care. The definitions for spiritual were widened (see Box 11.3). We subsequently found that the HIV/AIDS teams assessed the spiritual item much more frequently than the cancer teams.

The frequency of STAS assessments was reduced for HIV/AIDS patients. Patients were assessed at referral and then fortnightly (cancer, weekly) until discharge or death, unless there was a change in their circumstances. HIV/AIDS patients tend to spend longer in care than cancer patients (see Box 11.2) (mean time in care HIV/AIDS: 16 weeks CCT/41 weeks HST, cancer: 7 weeks)[1,3]. Their health and circumstances may also remain relatively stable for many weeks and during these times there may be very little contact with the team.

Box 11.3: Revised ratings for spiritual

0 = Content in self and world view, without feelings of guilt or punishment over illness. Any denomination or agnostic.
1 = Occasional doubts or unrealistic expectations. Patient able to resolve their feelings/problems themselves.
2 = Uncertain, sometimes troubled. Doubts. Patients unable to resolve their feelings/problems themselves.
3 = Uncertain and guilty. For example, troubled, conflicts, worry.
4 = Distraught with uncertainty or guilt over beliefs. In chaos as to how to remedy situation. Crisis, unable to resolve things, inability to cope, symptomatic (physical/emotional).

Other modifications

The teams record whether or not patients have a GP at referral and at death or discharge, and whether they are aware of the patients' diagnosis. They also record the involvement of district nurses, social workers, occupational therapists and volunteers at referral and death or discharge. HIV/AIDS patients tend to have a lower degree of GP (family doctor) involvement than cancer patients and one of the teams' roles is to increase the involvement of other professionals in HIV/AIDS patients' care[1,4].

The HIV/AIDS teams were keen to record the number of hours spent on home visits whereas the cancer teams had only recorded the number of home visits carried out. Due to the lower level of GP involvement and the smaller numbers of HIV/AIDS patients in care, the HIV/AIDS teams originally provided a great deal of 'hands on' care and they felt that it was important to assess the level of input (ie time) per patient.

Additional information collected by CCT

The CCT assessed an additional item, team anxiety, and also developed their own audit items to assess patients' individual symptoms.

Audit of HIV/AIDS teams

The evaluation of the CCT and HST considered patient characteristics, the audit of care using STAS, and inverviews with a sample of patients and carers at home (revalidation of STAS)

Methods

Teams collected data on all patients referred and remaining in care until discharge or death, the HST from May 1988 for 25 months, the CCT from July 1988 for 31 months. Patients were assessed according to the STAS at referral and then fortnightly until their discharge or death when a final assessment was made.

Results

Patient characteristics
During the study period 234 (116 HST, 118 CCT) patients were referred to the teams, of which 203 died in care, 12 were re-admitted and died in care, 18 were discharged and one committed suicide. Most patients were male (232), mean age 37.9 years (range 21–61), and most were homosexual (197) or bi-sexual (28).

| Place of care | At referral | | At death | |
	HST (n = 88)* n (%)	CCT (n = 100)* n (%)	HST (n = 108) n (%)	CCT (n = 105) n (%)
Home	29 (33)	54 (54)	22 (20)	31 (30)
Hospital	58 (66)	40 (40)	75 (69)	38 (36)
Hospice	1 (1)	6 (6)	11 (10)	36 (34)

* Recording of place of care at referral was introduced during the study Missing: At death place of care was not recorded for one HST and one CCT patient

Table 11.1: Place of care at referral and at death

Most patients were referred from hospital ward rounds or nurses, or from genitourinary clinics. Most common reasons for referral were: HST – symptom control (31%), patient support (28%) and patient anxiety (24%); and CCT – symptom control (68%) and home support (25%).

Patients spent significantly longer in the care of the HST. Median time in care for the HST was 42 weeks (range 0 to 115 weeks) and for the CCT 9.5 weeks (range 0 to 68 weeks). Median time from referral to death was for the HST 43 weeks and for the CCT 11 weeks.

Place of care at referral and at death are shown in Table 11.1. Common main symptoms at referral and death are shown in Figures 11.1 and 11.2.

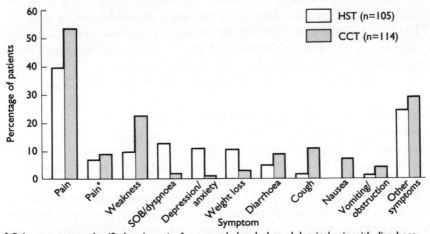

* Other symptoms classified under pain, for example headaches, abdominal pain with diarrhoea, pain from a wound or pressure sore

Figure 11.1: Main symptoms at referral

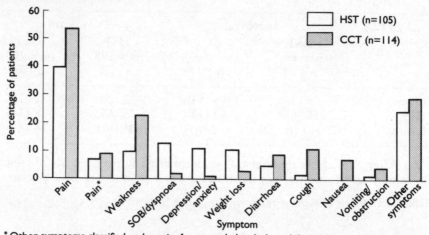

* Other symptoms classified under pain, for example headaches, abdominal pain with diarrhoea,
pain from a wound or pressure sore

Figure 11.2: Main symptoms at death

Audit data

STAS ratings identified symptom control, patient anxiety and family
anxiety as the most common severe problems for patients in the care of
both teams, at referral and throughout care until their death. Differences
between the teams were identified[1]. At referral, ratings for CCT patients were significantly more severe than those for HST patients. For
both teams the percentage of patients with severe ratings (ie 3 or 4) for
family anxiety increased slightly as the week of death approached.

Figures 11.3 and 11.4 show the percentage of patients with ratings of
3 and 4 (indicating severe problems) for symptom control and family
anxiety at referral, two weeks after referral (referral +2), two weeks
before death (death −2) and at death, for all patients who died in care.

Revalidation of STAS with HIV/AIDS patients

To allow STAS to be revalidated with HIV/AIDS patients, independent
assessments of STAS items for both patients and carers in the care of one
team (CCT) were made[5].

Nineteen patients and eight carers were interviewed, at home, three to
four weeks after referral. There was reasonable agreement and few differences between patient, carer and team assessments (Wilcoxon Z range
0.00 to −2.45) suggesting that the audit is valid and that providers'
views of care are a reasonable record of patient and carer experiences.
However, patients' assessments of pain were significantly more severe
than the teams' (p < 0.05, Wilcoxon Z −2.45)[5].

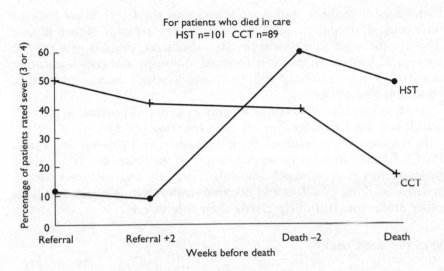

Figure 11.3: Symptom control: percentage of patients rated severe (3 or 4)

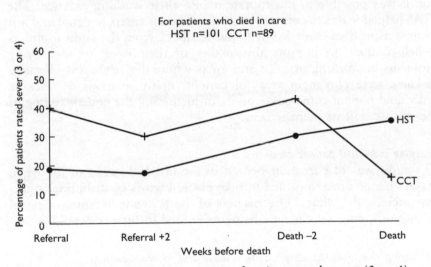

Figure 11.4: Family anxiety: percentage of patients rated severe (3 or 4)

Patients and carers made negative comments about communication, discussion of diagnosis and prognosis with professionals other than the team and lack of clarification as to the team's role in care[5].

Feedback

The results of the audit have been fed back to the teams and have led to improvements to their working practice. For example, the audit highlighted a problem with later referrals to the CCT. Many patients were being referred to the team in crisis at a very late stage of their illness. This led the team to review their referral criteria, develop new referral forms and leaflets, to consider their relationships and communication with other professionals, and to provide, where necessary, further education and advice.

STAS ratings identified family anxiety as a serious problem at referral, which had not been identified by staff referring patients.

In response to the feedback from interviews with patients and carers the CCT have carried out a separate study of their patients, asking them to assess their pain, at weekly intervals. They also reviewed their referral criteria, working practices and communication with patients and with other professionals, to help clarify their role in care.

Was the audit useful?

The HIV/AIDS teams found STAS useful in clarifying areas of their work and it was possible to incorporate it into their working practice. The STAS helped teams to consider patients and their carers in detail and not to miss aspects of care. Teams found feedback from the audit useful as it helped them to improve the quality of their work by identifying problems in working practice and areas where they were less effective.

There were two main areas of benefit, firstly in terms of tracking individual patient care and secondly in furthering the understanding of the disease and its management.

Tracking individual patient care

The audit was of particular benefit in the last few weeks of life when major change often appeared to take place. Factors contributing to this may include the clinical effectiveness of the teams in symptom control or interventions. This is now being examined in further detail.

Furthering the understanding of the disease and its management

The data collected showed the diversity and severity of symptoms experienced. For example, breathlessness and neurological problems were identified as being difficult to control and as the main determinants of hospital deaths. The influence of psychosocial factors on both patient and family choice of place of death was also identified. These findings suggest more commonality between palliative care for the HIV/AIDS and cancer patients than was anticipated five years ago.

As with cancer patients[6], symptom control and family anxiety remained severe problems for many patients at death. Audit could be used to study the control of individual symptoms in greater detail and to identify those which are particularly difficult for teams to control.

The adapted STAS works equally well with both cancer and HIV/AIDS patients to provide information on their problems and needs and the effectiveness of services.

References

1 Butters E, Higginson I, Wade A, McCarthy M, George R and Smits A (1991) Community HIV/AIDS teams. *Health Trends* **23**(2): 59–62.

2 George R (1991) *Care of people with HIV in the community: the experience of the Bloomsbury Community Care Team.* The All Parliamentary Group on AIDS, occasional paper number 2.

3 Ward A (1985) *Home care services for the terminally ill: a report for the Nuffield Foundation.* Sheffield: Medical Research Unit, Sheffield University.

4 Smits A, Mansfield S and Singh S (1990) Facilitating care of patients with HIV infection by hospital and primary care teams. *British Medical Journal* **300**: 241–3.

5 Butters E, Higginson I, George R and McCarthy M (1993) Palliative care for people with HIV/AIDS: views of patients, carers and providers. *AIDS Care* **5**(1): 105–16.

6 Higginson I, Wade A and McCarthy M (1992) Effectiveness of two palliative support teams. *Journal of Public Health Medicine* **14**(1): 50–6.

Further reading

Butters E, Higginson I, George R, Smits A and McCarthy M (1992(a)) Assessing the symptoms, anxiety and practical needs of HIV/AIDS patients receiving palliative care. *Quality of Life Research* **1**(1): 47–51.

Butters E, Higginson I, George R and McCarthy M (1992(b)) *A comparison of two quality of life measures in HIV/AIDS patients receiving palliative care.* In Poster abstracts book, PuB 3562, pp. B180. VIIIth International Conference on AIDS/IIIrd STD World Congress, Amsterdam, July, 1992.

George R (1990) Care of patients with late stage HIV infection and AIDS. *Cancer Care* **17**, Issue 1.

Hays R and Shapiro M (1992) An overview of generic health-related quality of life measure for HIV research. *Quality of Life Research* **1**(2): 91–7.

Higginson I (1990) *Evaluation of care for HIV/AIDS patients by two community teams in London, UK*. Report commissioned by the Regional Programme for AIDS, World Health Organization, Copenhagen.

McCarthy M and Higginson I (1991) Clinical audit by a palliative care team. *Palliative Medicine* 5(3): 29–35.

Pye M, Kapila M, Buckley G and Cunningham D (eds) (1989) *Responding to the AIDS challenge. A comparative study of local AIDS programmes in the United Kingdom*. Harlow: Longman.

Sims R and Moss V (1991) *Terminal care for people with AIDS*. London: Edward Arnold.

Watchel T, Piette J, Mor V, Stein M, Fleishman, J and Carpenter C (1992) Quality of life in persons with human immunodeficiency virus infection: measurement by the Medical Outcomes Study instrument. *Annals of Internal Medicine* 116(2): 131–7.

12

Audit Methods. Palliative Care: Guidelines for Good Practice and Audit Measures

(Report of a working group of the Research Unit, Royal College of Physicians)

Introduction

Palliative care is the active total care for patients whose disease is incurable. Control of pain, of other symptoms, and of psychological, social and spiritual problems is paramount. The goal of palliative care is achievement of the best possible quality of life for patients and their families[1,2].

Palliative care is a multidisciplinary activity taking place in Britain in a variety of settings – hospital wards under the aegis of symptom control teams, palliative care units, or at home with a specialized team advising the GP and the domiciliary nursing service.

Palliative medicine has recently been recognized as a specialty in the United Kingdom. Specialist medical training is available in centres which are approved for the purpose by the Joint Committee on Higher Medical Training. A requirement of such training is that audit measures are in place. This applies also to specialist nurse training. Since palliative care is a multi-professional activity, audit must also be multi-professional[3,4].

In order to develop and test constructive forms of audit, the Research Unit of the Royal College of Physicians in association with the Association for Palliative Medicine invited a multi-professional group to propose guidelines for good practice in palliative care in specialized in-patient units, and to propose audit measures whereby it might be seen whether that good practice was regularly achieved. The Working Group included representatives from medicine, nursing, social work, psychology, sociology, and a quality assurance consultant. Six background papers had been commissioned before the meeting on particular areas of interest and concern, as indicated by the headings in the text (*see* page 119). Circulation of these before the meeting allowed plenty of time for discussion, during which these guidelines were agreed.

Background

The characteristics of palliative care have been identified as attention to the whole needs of the individual, and the relief of symptoms whether physical, mental, spiritual or psychosocial. Care extends beyond patients to their families. Common features are bereavement support, and the continuing education and training of professionals and those volunteers who are also deployed in meeting the needs of the patient and his or her family. Emphasis on the quality of life remaining for the individual, good communication between and among patients, families and staff, and strong multi-professional teamwork are also features of palliative care.

Some of the endpoints of palliative care may be difficult to assess in the context of audit. A peaceful or dignified death may mean one thing to patients and families, and yet another to staff. The way in which bad news is conveyed may have a crucial effect not only on the feelings of patients and families, but also on how they cope with dying and death. The Research Unit of the Royal College of Physicians has previously tried to ensure that published guidelines for good practice (eg [5]) are supported by published scientific evidence of effectiveness. In the case of palliative care, such scientific evidence is harder to find. The guidelines are the product of the experience of a number of colleagues coming from different disciplines concerned with the care of the dying, and reflect the emotional, ethical and practical needs of the patients, their family and of those who work in palliative care units.

These guidelines are to help doctors by providing an analytical framework for the evaluation and treatment of some common clinical problems. They are not intended to replace a doctor's clinical judgement, and are not necessarily the only way in which a particular condition can be managed. They do, however, provide a framework within which audit and review of clinical practice can take place. The guidelines reflect the views of the individual clinicians who attended the workshops.

Guidelines

Admission to a palliative care unit: the first 24 hours

Before admission

- Whenever possible, contact should be made with the patient and/or relatives before admission to reduce fears. The reason for admission should be clearly stated in the case notes. The admission procedure should be documented in a nursing standard and should be explained to new team members.

On admission

- The patient should be examined by a doctor within two hours of arrival.
- After a brief initial assessment of symptoms[6], a medical, nursing and other care plan should be completed, preferably with a doctor and nurse working together for some of the admission procedure. The plan should be recorded in the case records.

After admission

- It is essential that the patient and family have opportunities to express their feelings and needs, and to seek information. The family should be offered a meeting with one or two of the team members.
- The patient will need to be orientated to his or her new environment. He or she should be introduced to the other patients, shown the facilities, and have the routines of the palliative care unit explained.
- The first meal is an opportunity to demonstrate individualized care, and the patient should be asked about his or her special dietary requirements.
- On the first evening he or she should be introduced personally to the night staff.
- The patient's symptoms and problems should be reassessed the day after admission. He or she may need to be introduced to other team members.

Quality of the environment in a palliative care unit

The Working Group did not consider basic administrative aspects such as the security with which drugs are stored and dispensed, and precautions against fire.

The *physical environment* needs regular assessment by a small group of lay people with a special interest in hospice care, as well as by senior staff working in the hospice. The assessment should include:

- cleanliness, decor, comfort and privacy
- the facilities for bathing and toileting, and for hairdressing, crafts and other diversional activities.

Assessment should also include:

- the quality of the catering
- control of noise and of smoking
- practical aspects such as the promptness with which the telephone is answered.

The *staff establishment* should be adequate to fulfil the care outlined in these guidelines. A Delphi exercise was conducted between 1986 and 1988 and some standards and guidelines for inpatient units were produced[7].

The *psychosocial environment* is also important. Staff should be friendly and efficient and accessible to patients and relatives. They should respond quickly to questions that worry patients or relatives.

Expectations of the patients receiving care

The clinical and ethical value of including the expectations of patients and caring relatives in auditing palliative care outweighs the disadvantages of imprecise assessment. Recording patients' expectations encourages and indicates clinical perceptiveness. The expectations of patients and their relatives may be inconsistent and affected by emotions and inexperience, but they are often rational and pertinent.

The clinical records relating to identified problems should include the expectations of patients and their relatives and the proposed professional action. Realistic expectations may reinforce or modify management. Expectations causing or threatening distress merit the record of a plan to help the patient or relative to adjust. Unfounded expectations that comfort the patient or his carer should be noted, with proposed actions or inaction. Subsequent records should state if the plans were enacted and, if not, why not. They should also record subsequent changes in expectations.

Communication to the patient and his or her relatives[8]

A palliative care unit should have a policy for communicating facts and opinions between professionals.

Traditional measures of successful communication in health care have been concerned with outcomes following information given to the patient, and with patient compliance. Neither of these is appropriate in palliative care as not all patients wish for information. Denial is one mechanism for coping. Informed choice is more important than compliance.

Research concerned with measuring the communication skills of health professionals suggests that much work is needed in this area to improve health care. Effective assessment of the problems of patients and their relatives will lead to care being based on their actual needs rather than those assumed. Patients should be asked whether they feel able to communicate their changing needs.

Successfully addressing the problems identified on admission

A recent study has shown that the most severe problems on admission are control of symptoms and family anxiety. Significant improvements in relief of patient symptoms after intervention by a hospice team can be demonstrated by the Support Team Assessment Schedule[9], but this study showed that family anxiety proved difficult to relieve, and although ratings improved initially, anxiety and other problems recurred at death. The Support Team Assessment Schedule enables team members to examine their work in more detail and to demonstrate the effectiveness of care.

Are those working in palliative care units able to deliver good care?

A palliative care unit should have written policies and procedures which ensure that access is not inadvertently denied to particular groups, eg those requiring admission within 24 hours of referral, or those of lower socio-economic status. A palliative care unit should use some broad measures of patient dependency. Such measures are being piloted in some areas, and are likely to prove to be a helpful tool.

Each palliative care unit should encourage and record the extent of formal and informal staff support and training, the rate of turnover of staff and sickness absence.

Audit measures

Admission policy

1. Are the different social groups in the catchment area of the hospice or specialized unit reflected proportionately in those admitted?
2. Is there a written policy about admissions, particularly in regard to those requiring urgent admission?
3. Is there a record of the reason for admission?
4. Is there a record of the waiting time before admission?
5. Is there a record of the main problems on admission?

Clinical management

6. Is there a record of previous problems and how they were treated?
7. Is there a record about the patient's pain, or was a pain chart completed at first assessment?

8. Is there a record of the patient's aims, expectation and objectives for each of his or her main problems?
9. Is there a record of an action plan and its outcome for each of the patient's main problems?
10. Is there a record of what happened to the patient in the first 24 hours after admission?
11. Were the action plans carried out or, if not, is there a record of the reasons for change?

Support of patients and relatives

12. Is there in place some system for monitoring the effectiveness of care such as the Support Team Assessment Schedule?
13. Is there a record of the patient's key relatives and their aims and expectations for each of the patient's main problems?
14. Is there a record of whether and how the expectations of patients and relatives were met or modified?
15. Is there a record of the health and coping strategies of the principal carer or relative?
16. Is there a record of the availability of home resources?

Communication

17. Is communication of facts between professionals carried out according to agreed policies?
18. Are patients asked whether they feel able to communicate their changing needs?
19. Is there a record of these changing needs, and are these needs addressed?
20. Are problems of communication within families recognized and appropriate steps taken?

Documentation and administration

21. Do the records contain a final discharge or death summary?
22. Is there a record of the patient's degree of dependency in the hospice or in-patient unit?
23. Is the staff establishment adequate for the needs of the patients admitted? (*See* reference[6] and background paper (f))
24. Is there regular appraisal of staff linked to in-service and extra-mural training opportunities?
25. What support system exists for staff and are individual members aware of it? (Suggested questions to staff are available in background paper (b))

26. Is there a record of and regular review of staff absence and sickness rates?
27. Is there a record of satisfaction of patients and their carers with care? (Suggested questions available in background paper (c))
28. Is there a record of the views of a visiting team about the quality of the environment in the units, from the perspective of patients, carers and staff? (Suggested points to be checked available in background papers (b) and (f))
29. Is there a record of all audit meetings, the names of those attending them, the decisions reached, the name of the person nominated to enable necessary change, and a date for a review of the problems encountered at audit?

Acknowledgements

The Research Unit of the Royal College of Physicians is supported by generous grants from the Wolfson and Welton Foundation, by other charitable donations, and by a grant from the Department of Health.

Background papers

The background papers prepared by some members of the Working Group (*listed below*) are available from the Publications Department, Royal College of Physicians, 11 St Andrews Place, London NW1 4LE, on payment of £6.00 for the set to cover costs of photocopying and postage. The Guidelines are available in soft cover, price £5.00.

a. What should happen in the first 24 hours after the admission to a hospice? By *P Kaye* and *J Phillips*
b. How do we measure the quality of the environment and autonomy of the patient in the hospice environment? By *E Wilkes*
c. The expectations of the patients receiving care, and whether these expectations are met. By *J Hinton*
d. How do we measure whether the communication to the patient and his relatives has been successful? By *Ann Faulkner*
e. How do we measure whether we have successfully addressed the problems identified on admission? By *Irene Higginson*
f. Are those working in palliative medicine able to deliver good care? By *Anne Naysmith*

References

1 Saunders C (ed.) (1985) *The management of terminal malignant diseases.* London: Arnold.

2 European Association for Palliative Care (1989) *Newsletter* No. 1.

3 Ford G (1990) Constructive audit. *Palliative Medicine* 4(1): Editorial.

4 Hopkins A (1990) *Measuring the quality of medical care.* London: RCP Publications.

5 Working Group of Research Unit of Royal College of Physicians (1991) Guidelines for the management of urinary infections in childhood. *Journal of the Royal College of Physicians London* 25: 36–42.

6 Hockley JM, Dunlop R and Davis R (1988) Survey of distressing symptoms in dying patients and their families in hospital and the response to a symptom control team. *British Medical Journal* 296: 1715–7.

7 Harper R, Ward A, Westlake L and Williams BT (1988) *Good practice in terminal care.* Department of Community Medicine, University of Sheffield Medical School.

8 Maguire P and Faulkner A (1988) How to do it: improve the counselling skills of doctors and nurses in cancer care. *British Medical Journal* 297: 847–8 and 972–4.

9 McCarthy M and Higginson IJ (1991) Clinical audit by a palliative care team. *Palliative Medicine* 5(3): 215–21.

Further reading

Higginson IJ, Wade JM and McCarthy M (1992) Effectiveness of two palliative support teams. *Journal of Public Health Medicine* 14(1): 50–6.

Acknowledgement

The text for this chapter was previously published in the *Journal of the Royal College of Physicians of London* (1991) 25(4): 325–8 and is reproduced with the kind permission of the editor of that journal.

13

Audit Methods: Analysing Results

IRENE HIGGINSON

Introduction

Frequent analysis of audit data is essential to complete the audit loop to maintain interest and enthusiasm (*see* Chapter 3). This chapter covers some basic pointers for those wishing to analyse and present audit data.

Many audits will begin without statistical analysis of data, because the unit will be identifying problems or suggesting changes, but at a later stage changes in practice and a more advanced audit may require further analysis. The further reading includes textbooks which give full details of the tests described here, and which give a comprehensive review of statistical methods.

Two components of analysing results

Analysing results has two components – data processing, which includes any statistical analysis, and interpretation of the results. These aspects are interdependent and should be seen as activities that go hand-in-hand rather than as separate stages[1]. When analysing data from clinical audit the amount of data is usually modest and it is straight-forward to first process the available information and then to interpret the results. In larger analyses it is important to analyse one set of results, consider these and then, seeing what inferences might be drawn from them and what further questions might emerge, decide what further analyses are needed. Trying in one go to ask everything you might possibly want to analyse can waste a lot of time.

Data processing

In many audits, it is perfectly possible to process the data without using a computer. Indeed, in the early stages of audit, when information on only a small number of patients is being collected, it is probably more sensible not to use a computer or to develop a data base (*see* Chapter 17 for more details). If a computer is used or if information is abstracted from notes and handwritten onto forms, it is very important to ensure that any coding is done correctly and there are no mistakes when transcribing and entering data onto a computer. A minimal useful check is a simple count – data have a nasty habit of going astray. Another is to check that none of the values of variables fall outside acceptable ranges; for example, a person aged 242 years, a person with a rating for pain or another problem that is outside the acceptable range, a person who was discharged before they were referred. If a computer is used it is possible to programme many of the packages or data bases to accept only valid values or to give a warning if a value is possibly wrong, for example if the date of admission is old.

To guide the analysis many researchers prepare, in advance, a skeleton table or figure, which indicates the types of analysis required and the questions to be answered. No hard and fast rules are laid down for the sequence of analysis but a generally advised order is shown in Box 13.1.

Box 13.1: Advised sequence of analysis[1]

1. Examine each variable separately.
2. Examine pairs of variables.
3. Examine sets of three or more variables.

To examine each variable separately, frequency distributions can be used. For an example *see* Box 13.2.

Box 13.2: Example of pain control scores

Recordings were made using the STAS on 38 patients at referral.

Score		Number of patients	Percentage of recordings
0	None	3	7.9
1	Mild	4	10.5
2	Moderate	8	21.1
3	Severe	12	31.6
4	Very severe	9	23.7
9	Unknown	2	5.3
Total		38	100.0

Valid number = 36   Missing = 2

The frequency distribution shows how many individuals fall into each category. At this stage it includes the number in the unknown or missing category. If there is a large number of individuals in the unknown or missing category, it may mean that this variable cannot be studied further. In audit, finding a large amount of missing information can indicate a need to improve documentation or assessment (*see* Chapters 5 and 7). The total number plus the number of any excluded from the analysis is given, so that the reader can get an idea of the size of the sample.

Graphs

The aim of a graph is to assist the reader to grasp the meaning of a series of numbers by means of the eye[2]. Graphs should be regarded as subsidiary aids to intelligence and *not* as evidence of association or trends[2]. That evidence should be drawn from the statistical tables and tests themselves. A graph or trend can be made to appear very different by changing the axis used. Figures 13.1 and 13.2 were drawn from the same data on the number of patients with severe anxiety in week 1 through to week 4 of care. Figure 13.1 axis starts at 0 and goes up to the total number of patients in care (38). This figure suggests only a slight reduction in the number of people with severe anxiety. In

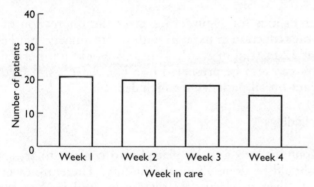

Figure 13.1: Number of patients with severe anxiety

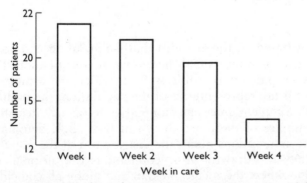

Figure 13.2: Number of patients with severe anxiety (different axis)

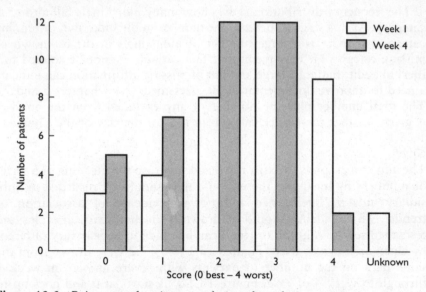

Figure 13.3: Pain control ratings: week 1 and week 4

contrast, the different axis for Figure 13.2 gives the impression of a marked decline in the reduction in patients with severe anxiety, but here the axis is ended at 12 instead of zero[2]. This axis would not normally be acceptable. Data can also be presented in a bar chart, as in Figure 13.3, where the data on all patients are included.

Interpretation of findings

Once a result is found it needs to be placed into context to try and understand what should be done about the finding. There are several questions which can help to clarify interpretation, and lead to conclusions and action (*see* Box 13.3).

Statistical anlaysis
Statistical analysis is based on the key idea that we make observations on a sample of patients or subjects and then draw inferences about the population of all such patients or subjects from which the sample is drawn. If the sample is not representative of the population, the finding may be misleading[3]. Simple indices can summarize frequency distributions and some examples of these are shown in Box 13.4. Summary statistics often make assumptions about the distribution of the population from which they are drawn. Most common is the 'normal' or Gaussian distribution where the mean, median and mode all coincide, the distribution is symmetrical about the mean and where nearly one

Box 13.3: Questions to consider when interpreting results in audit

Strength of finding – how much difference is there between groups, what is the statistical power, sample size?

Consistency of findings – have others found this also or are their findings opposite?

Clinical relevance – what does the finding mean to clinical practice, what differences could be made?

Plausibility – is the finding plausible and, if not, why? Does it support any anecdotal evidence or impressions, or act against these?

Bias – what possible bias may have affected the sample chosen, the recording of information, and how would these alter the results?

Conclusion – having answered these questions what does the finding mean to our clinical practice?

Action – what should be done now? Are there new standards we should set to repeat the audit cycle? Could we perform the audit in a better way next time, which would remove some of the bias?

Box 13.4: Some summary statistics

Mean – the average, the sum of all observations divided by the number of observations.

Median – the value or magnitude of the central or middle observation when all the observations are listed in order from lowest to highest. The median divides the distribution into two halves.

Mode – the most frequently occurring value in the series.

Standard deviation (SD) – a measure of the scatter of observations around their mean. It is determined by calculating difference between each of the variables and the mean (the deviation), squaring each of these, so there are no longer any negative values and then averaging them. (This value is known as the variance.) The standard deviation is the square root of this value.

Standard error (SE) of the mean – a measure of the uncertainty of the mean. In a single sample the standard error equals the standard deviation divided by the square root of the number in the sample (ie $SE = SD/\sqrt{n}$, where n = number in the sample). The standard error is used to calculate a confidence interval.

Confidence interval (*see* text for discussion) for a population mean is given by:

$$\text{mean} - (t_{i-a/2} \times SE) \text{ to mean} + (t_{i-a/2} \times SE)$$

Box 13.4: *Continued*

where $t_{i-a/2}$ is the appropriate value from the t distribution with
n − 1 degrees of freedom associated with a 'confidence' of
$100(1-a)\%$. For a 95% confidence interval a = 0.05. Values of t
can be found in statistical textbooks. However, an easy figure to
remember is that for a 95% confidence interval the value of $t_{i-a/2}$
will be close to 2 for samples of 20 upwards, but noticeably greater
than 2 for smaller samples.

---

third of the values will differ from the mean by more than once the
standard deviation and only about five per cent will differ by more than
twice the standard deviation. 'Parametric' statistical tests, such as a
t-test to measure differences between two groups, have been calculated
assuming that the data is normally distributed. Non-parametric tests,
such as the Mann Whitney U test or Wilcoxon Rank Sum test, can be
used if the data is not sufficiently close to a normal distribution[4].

Confidence intervals
Results from any single sample are subject to statistical uncertainty,
because of random variation. The degree of uncertainty is strongly
related to the size of the sample. Confidence intervals indicate the
precision or imprecision of the study sample estimates as population
values. During the 1980s some studies in scientific journals were
criticized because the results were presented in terms of levels of sig-
nificance, with no mention of actual concentrations or proportions or
their differences. Clearly such information is needed to indicate the
clinical importance of any statistical difference. A confidence interval
provides a move from a single value estimate, such as a mean, median,
proportion or correlation, to a range of values that are considered to be
plausible to the population. The width of a confidence interval associated with a sample statistic depends partly on its standard error (*see*
Box 13.4) and hence of the scatter of the observations and the sample
size. It also depends on the degree of 'confidence' to be associated with
the resulting interval. For example, if the mean level of pain is 2.4 and
the 95% confidence interval ranges from 1.4 to 3.4, this indicates that
if a series of identical studies were carried out repeatedly in 95 out of
100, the mean level of pain would be found to be between 1.4 and 3.4.
Full details on the calculation of confidence intervals can be found in
Gardner and Altman[3], and many statistical packages. One calculation
is shown in Box 13.4.

Conclusions

Analysis consists of two stages: data processing and interpretation of the findings. Processing audit data will normally require fairly straight-forward examination of data beginning with single variables and then progressing to examining one variable at different times or two variables. To interpret findings a series of questions about the strength, consistency, clinical relevance, plausibility and possible biases can help, and lead to conclusions and a plan of action. To be sure that differences found between variables measured at different times have not occurred by chance, more complicated statistical analysis is needed, to determine the confidence of the findings.

References

1 Abramson JH (1990) *Survey methods in community medicine.* Epidemiological studies, programme evaluation, clinical trials (4th edition). Edinburgh: Churchill Livingstone.

2 Hill AB (1977) *A short textbook of medical statistics.* London: Hodder and Stoughton.

3 Gardner MJ and Altman DG (1989) Statistics with confidence – confidence intervals and statistical guidelines. London: British Medical Journal.

4 Bland M (1987) *An introduction to medical statistics.* Oxford: Oxford University Press.

Further reading

Altman D (1991) *Practical statistics for medical research.* London: Chapman and Hall.

14

Audit Experience: A Nurse Manager in Home Care

ELIZABETH McKEE

Introducing audit to our hospice has been a worthwhile investment. The home care team are now very familiar with it and include it as an integral part of their work. The introduction of audit has been a slower process in the in-patient unit as it was running alongside other major changes such as primary nursing. It meant that the medical staff took responsibility for the scoring which is not entirely satisfactory if a multi-disciplinary approach to care is being accepted. However, over the past couple of months, the audit scores have become part of the weekly multidisciplinary ward round. It is early days to assess the value of this approach but other disciplines are now having the opportunity to comment. Inevitably the ward meetings have become longer and we are now looking at how the time can be used more effectively. The home care team continues to score the patients on their caseload on a weekly basis, with each home care sister taking responsibility for his/her own caseload.

Did we need audit?

Quality assurance and audit are current buzz words in industry, education and health care. The organization I work for is a hospice within the voluntary sector. For us too, quality assurance and audit have become important issues. Local health boards buying in palliative care services from the hospice want to make sure they are getting value for money and the best possible service.

In some ways we have had a fool's pardon since we opened in 1985. Everyone assumed that hospice care was of a high standard, perhaps due to a wave of enthusiasm that swept through the United Kingdom as hospice units and home care teams mushroomed in number. It is now no longer good enough to say we practise good quality care. We have to be able to prove that we do.

The management of the hospice recognized that we had to find some way of auditing the care we were giving to dying patients and their families. We thus entered into the first step of introducing audit – which was recognizing a need for it.

Choosing a system of audit

The second stage was to find out how to do it. Several models of audit were looked at in an attempt to find one that would suit the needs of the hospice unit. Box 14.1 summarizes what we were looking for.

After a time of reading and investigation we were most interested in the Support Team Assessment Schedule (STAS)[1]. We made contact with the authors who supplied the most recent information on STAS.

Box 14.1: Requirements for audit

1. Simple to use.
2. Tried and tested package.
3. Not too time consuming.
4. A 'believable' package.

Planning for audit

The third stage involved setting up a small working group which consisted of two medical staff and myself. This group's point of reference was to adapt the STAS system to our own needs. Each of the definitions listed by Higginson (*see* Chapter 5) were looked at and discussed to determine their relevance to our unit. We decided that we did not want to initially score two items: 'predictability' and 'planning', so these were omitted. We did, however, want to broaden the definitions for symptom control. The original STAS defines symptom control under 'other symptom control' which we felt was limiting. We therefore identified 13 common symptoms experienced in palliative care (listed in Box 14.2) which we felt would be worth further scrutiny.

We then set about writing the scoring definitions, adhering closely to the format used in the STAS. We consulted closely with Dr Higginson to ensure that we were not straying from the original format and wording. Dr Higginson also met with the working group to help us

---

Box 14.2: List of items added to the STAS (*see* Appendix B)

1. Nausea
2. Vomiting
3. Oral problems
4. Dysphagia
5. Dyspnoea
6. Anorexia
7. Pruritus

8. Constipation
9. Diarrhoea
10. Cough
11. Haemoptysis
12. Lymphoedema
13. Pressure sore/skin lesion

---

clarify our thinking on audit and to help us to understand more fully the STAS model. This was a very useful meeting when questions were answered and our thinking became more clear.

Getting staff involved

Introducing audit into the work situation means change for staff. An awareness of change management is, therefore, important if audit is to be introduced effectively.

Communication and consultation are particularly important in times of change. Mullins suggests that staff will accept change more readily if they have been consulted[2], *see* Box 14.3.

Box 14.3: Requirements for effective change[2]:

1. Fully inform staff of proposals.
2. Encourage a positive attitude.
3. Involve staff.
4. Shared commitment of staff.

From an early stage in our development of audit we tried to keep staff informed of what was happening. At staff meetings we discussed the need for audit and shared with staff how we were hoping to implement an audit package. The discussions were on the whole positive although they did raise some concerns (*see* Box 14.4) on which we were able to give reassurance.

Box 14.4: Concerns raised by staff

1. How much time is involved?
2. How much extra paperwork will be involved?
3. Will we see the results?
4. How will it benefit us?
5. Is it user friendly?

Once the paperwork had been completed and our new definitions were typed and ready for completion, we decided to organize a workshop on audit for the staff, and organized a facilitated day. The workshop day was very successful. The morning programme gave senior staff the opportunity to share and clarify the workings of STAS. The afternoon session helped to 'sell' STAS to staff in a very positive and meaningful way. The workshop reassured staff and it was helpful to see some results obtained from other units already using STAS. We divided the day as outlined in Box 14.5. At the end of the day staff left with a feeling of 'this is worth trying'.

Box 14.5: Programme for 'audit' workshop

1. Morning – informal discussion between Dr Higginson and the four staff members responsible for overseeing audit.
2. Afternoon – audit seminar for all clinical staff (in-patient unit, day care and home care); facilitator – Dr Higginson.

Programme – Why audit?
           – What is audit?
           – What is STAS and how to use it?
           – Discussion and questions.

Getting started

We had now reached the stage of actually 'doing' the audit. All the preparation and planning was completed, paperwork was ready and staff training had taken place. It was time to strike while the iron was hot so as not to lose any of the enthusiasm. Each staff member was given their own complete copy of the STAS definitions to make the process of scoring easier.

We started by scoring only new patients referred from the agreed start date. This introduced the audit gradually and it was about three months before every patient was being scored. Staff were therefore able to adjust gradually to the scoring. It was agreed to score on the date of the first visit and weekly thereafter. We also decided not to audit every variable on the form as we felt this could be taking on too much. Instead we scored the 12 original variables as identified by Higginson along with nausea, vomiting, oral problems, constipation and dyspnoea.

Staff quickly got to grips with STAS. There were some minor initial problems which were quickly resolved with discussion, *see* Box 14.6.

Box 14.6: Early problems we quickly resolved

- Learning to interpret the definitions.
- When to use a 'missing' score.
- How to add up scores.
- Getting the message across that scoring must reflect the patient's view of the problem.

Evaluation of audit

We have not, as yet, carried out a formal evaluation of our audit programme but already we can identify some of the benefits. The STAS model has been accepted by staff and has become an integral part of patient care. We think STAS is an appropriate model for audit for our unit at the present time. *See* Box 14.7 for a summary of identified benefits.

Box 14.7: Benefits of STAS

- User-friendly.
- Quick to complete.
- Clearly shows staff if patient symptoms and well-being are improving.
- Helps to identify problem areas and difficult symptoms.
- Encourages discussion regarding patient problems.
- Helps staff to identify if a change of approach to a specific problem is required.

Results

Another factor of successful audit is feedback. Staff will soon become disillusioned if they cannot see the results of their data collection and scoring. A computer programme is now available for use with STAS (*see* Chapter 17), courtesy of the Irish Cancer Society, which means that patient scores can be analysed very quickly and immediate results and feedback obtained. We obtained permission from the Irish Cancer Society to adapt this programme for an interface with our own clinical data base which enables us to transfer data between the two programmes without duplication. At the time of writing we are just about to begin using this programme. To date we have had to do a manual analysis of the results.

We found manual analysis of STAS scores relatively easy although it was time consuming as any manual analysis would be. Even though many units now have access to computers, it is useful to be aware that STAS can be of value whether a computer is available or not.

There follows a selection of tables illustrating some results obtained from an analysis of the first 84 patients referred to the home care team whose care we audited using STAS. The percentages shown in the tables are given as a percentage of those patients still alive at each week. It should be noted for example, that by week eight only 18 of the 84 patients were still alive. While this does have an influence on the results, it still shows clearly that improvements in symptoms could be measured. The dyspnoea scores were measured in the first 77 patients.

Tables 14.1 to 14.7 show a sample of individual symptoms which were scored. The tables show the combined scores on referral and after one week, two weeks, four weeks and eight weeks.

Table 14.1 shows the scores for pain control. It can be seen clearly that the scores reduced considerably after only one week and by week eight only 6% of patients scored had severe pain (score 3 or 4) as opposed to 21% on referral. Those patients with no pain (score 0) increased from 40% on referral to 72% at week eight. None of the patients had a score of 4, the most severe pain at week eight.

Table 14.2 showing the scores for constipation also indicates a good improvement. It was disturbing to find that 49% of patients had moderate to severe constipation (scores 2–4 and causing patient distress) on referral. Again, after only one week this had reduced to 24% and at week eight only 6% of patients had moderate constipation and 72% scored zero.

Weeks in care	n	Score 0	1	2	3	4	9
On referral	84	33 (40%)	11 (13%)	22 (26%)	13 (16%)	4 (5%)	1 (1%)
Week one	73	40 (55%)	19 (26%)	12 (16%)	2 (3%)	0	
Week two	58	33 (57%)	12 (21%)	9 (16%)	2 (3%)	2 (3%)	
Week four	40	25 (63%)	10 (25%)	3 (7%)	2 (5%)	0	
Week eight	18	13 (72%)	2 (11%)	2 (11%)	1 (6%)	0	

9 = missing score

Table 14.1: Percentage of patients with different pain control scores

Weeks in care	n	Score 0	1	2	3	4	9
On referral	84	33 (39%)	9 (11%)	26 (31%)	8 (10%)	7 (8%)	1 (1%)
Week one	73	38 (52%)	18 (24%)	13 (18%)	2 (3%)	2 (3%)	
Week two	58	26 (44%)	20 (35%)	8 (14%)	3 (5%)	1 (2%)	
Week four	40	19 (48%)	14 (35%)	5 (12%)	2 (5%)	0	
Week eight	18	13 (72%)	4 (22%)	1 (6%)	0	0	

9 = missing score

Table 14.2: Percentage of patients with different constipation scores

Weeks in care	n	Scores 0	1	2	3	4	9
On referral	84	52 (62%)	7 (8%)	11 (13%)	8 (10%)	5 (6%)	1 (1%)
Week one	73	55 (75%)	8 (11%)	5 (7%)	3 (4%)	2 (3%)	
Week two	58	39 (67%)	11 (19%)	5 (9%)	2 (3%)	1 (2%)	
Week four	40	27 (68%)	8 (20%)	3 (8%)	1 (2%)	0	1 (2%)
Week eight	18	15 (83%)	3 (6%)	0	0	0	

9 = missing score

Table 14.3: Percentage of patients with different nausea scores

Weeks in care	n	Score 0	1	2	3	4	9
On referral	84	60 (71%)	8 (10%)	6 (7%)	6 (7%)	3 (4%)	1 (1%)
Week one	73	59 (81%)	7 (10%)	3 (4%)	3 (4%)	1 (1%)	
Week two	58	49 (84%)	4 (7%)	4 (7%)	1 (2%)	0	
Week four	40	34 (85%)	2 (5%)	4 (10%)	0	0	
Week eight	18	17 (94%)	1 (6%)	0	0	0	

9 = missing score

Table 14.4: Percentage of patients with different vomitting scores

Weeks in care	n	Score 0	1	2	3	4	9
On referral	84	4 (5%)	18 (21%)	23 (27%)	21 (25%)	14 (17%)	4 (5%)
Week one	73	6 (8%)	27 (37%)	24 (33%)	10 (14%)	5 (7%)	1 (1%)
Week two	58	10 (17%)	20 (34%)	14 (24%)	12 (21%)	1 (2%)	1 (2%)
Week four	40	7 (17%)	14 (35%)	9 (23%)	4 (10%)	4 (10%)	2 (5%)
Week eight	18	3 (17%)	7 (39%)	6 (33%)	2 (11%)	0	

9 = missing score

Table 14.5: Percentage of patients with different anxiety scores

Weeks in care	n	Score 0	1	2	3	4	9
On referral	84	3 (4%)	11 (13%)	20 (24%)	21 (25%)	21 (25%)	8 (9%)
Week one	73	2 (3%)	21 (29%)	24 (33%)	10 (14%)	9 (12%)	7 (9%)
Week two	58	5 (9%)	16 (27%)	19 (33%)	7 (12%)	6 (10%)	5 (9%)
Week four	40	5 (13%)	11 (28%)	13 (32%)	6 (15%)	3 (7%)	2 (5%)
Week eight	18	3 (17%)	7 (39%)	6 (34%)	1 (5%)	0	1 (5%)

9 = missing score

Table 14.6: Percentage of families with different anxiety scores

Weeks in care	n	Score 0	1	2	3	4	9
On referral	77	38 (49%)	14 (18%)	13 (17%)	7 (9%)	4 (6%)	1 (1%)
Week one	66	34 (51%)	14 (21%)	9 (14%)	7 (11%)	2 (3%)	
Week two	51	28 (54%)	10 (20%)	7 (14%)	5 (10%)	1 (2%)	
Week four	34	19 (56%)	5 (15%)	6 (17%)	4 (12%)	0	
Week eight	18	10 (56%)	2 (11%)	3 (17%)	2 (11%)	0	1 (5%)

9 = missing score

Table 14.7: Percentage of patients with different dyspnoea scores

Table 14.3 shows the scores for nausea which can be one of the more difficult symptoms to score. It was encouraging to see that once again the scores reduced after one week and at eight weeks 83% of patients did not complain of nausea. The scores for vomiting, shown in Table 14.4 give a similar picture to that of the nausea scores.

Patient anxiety scores are displayed in Table 14.5 and again a general improvement in scores was evident. The scores for family anxiety are shown in Table 14.6 and while there was again an improvement in the scores it was of interest to note that the majority of families remained in the little anxiety to moderate anxiety (scores 1 – 3) categories. Those families who were extremely anxious (score 4) were 5% to 9% up until week four. This emphasized the need for good family support.

These results were certainly very encouraging and staff were able to see quite clearly that their input was indeed improving patient symptoms. STAS also helps to identify problem areas and we found that dyspnoea (shown in Table 14.7), was one of them. This would show a similarity to Higginson et al.[3] where dyspnoea was also identified as a symptom where scores did not improve significantly. Scores which do not reduce or scores which actually increase stimulate discussion in an attempt to improve the situation or to find a reason for the non-improvement. It has given staff the opportunity to examine in detail the care given to patients and their families. Sometimes a new approach will be identified which will subsequently reduce scores. Discussion can also show staff that it is sometimes difficult to add to the care already being given and, despite a high level of input from the team, scores for some patients can remain high. In these situations, staff can be reassured that they are doing their best as discussion did not identify any changes in care that should be made.

Conclusions

Box 14.8 summarizes the steps we took to introduce audit in what has proved to be a painless and worthwhile manner. We now look forward

---

Box 14.8: Step by step guideline to audit

1. Staff informed from the beginning.
2. Decision made as to which model.
3. Working group set up.
4. Audit model adapted to our needs.
5. Further staff discussion.
6. Staff training.
7. Some results fed back.

to transferring our audit scoring onto the computer which will give us much more detailed feedback and analysis. We hope that this will help us to further monitor our care and also to be able to prove that we are providing the best possible care for the dying patient and his or her family.

It is also clear that this has only been a start to the whole process of audit and quality assurance for us. We have much more to do and learn. However, our introduction to audit has been a positive experience and we must now act on the results and continue to move forward. We are already looking at tools for nursing audit to supplement the STAS audit in the in-patient unit.

References

1 McCarthy M and Higginson I (1991) Clinical audit by a palliative care team. *Palliative Medicine* 5(3): 215–21.

2 Mullins LJ (1989) *Management and organisational behaviour*, (2nd edition). London: Pitman. 504–5.

3 Higginson I and McCarthy M (1989) Measuring symptoms in terminal cancer: are pain and dyspnoea controlled? *Journal of the Royal Society of Medicine* 82: 264–7.

15

Audit Experience: Assessing Staff Views

ANNE HAYES

Introduction

Our Lady's Hospice was founded in 1879. It is a free-standing hospice incorporating two palliative care units with 42 beds and a home care team. Approximately 450 patients are cared for in the in-patient units and 300 by the home care team annually.

In March 1991 Our Lady's Hospice had its first meeting to consider the setting up of a clinical audit system. Medical, nursing and administrative staff attended this meeting which was facilitated by a physician experienced in audit.

Audit and how it relates to palliative care was discussed, helping to clarify and alleviate our many concerns and questions. The Support Team Assessment Schedule (STAS) was also introduced. The STAS had previously been used to assess patients and families and has been validated for use as a measure of aspects affecting quality of life. It is also known to have a high level of inter-rater reliability[1] (see Chapter 6).

Over the following months medical and nursing staff, representing both home care and in-patient palliative care teams, met to identify those areas of care which would be the focus for audit. Concurrent meetings were also set up for the nursing staff to introduce and familiarize them with STAS.

In July 1991, STAS was introduced in both the palliative care units and home care, to be completed on the admission (or first visit) of a patient, weekly thereafter and following the death of the patient. The items chosen for audit were seven patient and family items: pain control, other symptom control, patient anxiety, family anxiety, patient insight, family insight and communication between patient and family; and two service items: communication between professionals and communication from professionals to patient and family. The STAS is problem orientated and items are rated 0 to 4. Definitions for each item and each point are documented.

Reviewing STAS in September 1991, it was decided to develop and include four additional items: patient well-being (patient perspective), patient well-being (staff perspective), family well-being and staff anxiety (*see* Appendix C). One of the main reasons for this was the 'feeling' that it was difficult to rate pain and symptom control without getting a clearer picture of how the patient was in him or herself.

Twelve months after introducing STAS it was decided to evaluate the staff's experience to its introduction and use on a weekly basis. It is important to note that at the time of the evaluation the staff had not had an opportunity to view STAS in its wider context ie statistical analysis of the results over a period of time.

Method

During two days 25 questionnaires (*see* Appendix J) were distributed to nurses and doctors on both in-patient and home care palliative care teams in Our Lady's Hospice. Staff were asked to record anonymously, in open ended questions, their reaction to the introduction of clinical audit and their experience of using this audit system on a weekly basis. They described the most and least useful aspects and whether they wished to continue the audit system.

Results

Twenty-one completed questionnaires were returned (a response rate of 84%), 14 from in-patient staff and seven from home care staff. Table 15.1 indicates the staff's reaction to the introduction of the audit system.

Fifteen respondents indicated that the introductory meetings were useful because they 'allowed for open discussion' and 'clarification of the workings and uses of audit', thereby giving an insight into what could be achieved. It was also suggested that having an introductory meeting made it 'a team approach'. Of the remaining respondents, three were not employed by Our Lady's Hospice at the time of its introduction.

Table 15.2 indicates the staff's opinion of the usefulness of the audit system at the time of evaluation.

Further comments included, that using STAS helps to 'identify problems' and 'decide on priorities'. It was also seen as a 'useful measure of pain and symptom control', giving 'an overall picture of the patient on admission and how pain and other symptoms are managed and

Response	Number
Good idea	12
Might be useful	4
Unsure	–
More work for the nurses	2
More paperwork	2
More change	–
Complicated	1
Of no use	–

Table 15.1: Reaction to the introduction of audit (n = 21)

Response	Number
Useful	15
Unsure	1
Of no use	5

Table 15.2: Usefulness of audit system (n = 21)

Response	Number
Helps to identify problems	11
Helps to clarify problems	2
Helps to clarify what changes are taking place	
(i) for the patient	9
(ii) for the family	5
Gives overview of patients' progress	10
Quick and easy to complete	4
Other comments	–

Note: the numbers in these groups are not mutually exclusive as some respondents chose more than one category.

Table 15.3: Most useful aspects (n = 21)

Response	Number
Increased workload	6
Increased time	7
Another form to complete	6
Fails to show clear picture of patient	10
Not detailed enough	2

Note: some respondents chose more than one category.

Table 15.4: Least useful aspects (n = 21)

resolved'. The 'focus is as a ward team looking at a whole range of patient and family problems' and using STAS 'helps to refocus our aims and goals of care drawing attention to disimprovement quickly, efficiently and non-accusingly'. One respondent who was unsure of the usefulness of using STAS commented that 'it does not tell us anything new, summarizing what is already known, but it gives an overview of the patient's condition during the week'.

The reasons given by another respondent who did not find the audit system useful was that it was found to be inappropriate at times, for example when a patient is admitted who dies shortly afterwards.

Table 15.3 indicates the most useful aspects of STAS as identified by the staff.

Considering the least useful aspects of STAS (*see* Table 15.4) one respondent suggested that 'it gives medical pointers rather than a refined audit from the patients' perspective', and that the 'psychological status of the patient is unclear'.

Sixteen respondents considered it worthwhile continuing this method of audit. The reasons given were that this is a 'tried and tested method', helping to 'review and address weekly problems'. It 'also makes one think about how the patient and family are', and can serve to be a 'measure of the patient's condition'.

Five respondents did not consider it worthwhile continuing this method of audit, the main reason given was that it was 'time consuming'. One of the respondents also suggested that 'most of the questions' asked in order to complete the STAS 'have already been looked at, however, it is a useful tool to give an overview of the patient on admission'.

Modifications which the respondents would like to see introduced included:

- having the capacity to score each symptom separately
- development of the psychological well-being of the patient because 'there is no room to record where the patient is with regard to his/her level of acceptance of his/her disease/dying'
- clarify who the family members are. In STAS the family is taken as the patient's nearest carer but other family members may be or become involved which cannot be included at present
- clarification of whether staff should score a point in time, or an overview of the past week. There are inconsistencies in the way staff score STAS at present.

Discussion

The palliative care staff have found using STAS on a weekly basis to be useful in their practice, helping them to identify, prioritize and address problems. Both the in-patient and home care teams are also able to monitor and review problems more quickly and efficiently, identifying areas where they are effective and where aims of care have to be reviewed. Although problem-orientated, STAS is an holistic approach to measuring care, and the focus is as a multidisciplinary team considering each patient and family on a weekly basis.

It is interesting to note, however, that while problems may be identified, ten respondents suggested that it fails to show a clear picture of the patient. This may be due to our difficulty in measuring the qualitative aspects of care. STAS ratings record the staff's perceptions of patient and family needs. To help overcome this we introduced a new item entitled 'patient well-being' which was to be rated directly by the patient. The main advantage of this is that the patient is more involved and it is also a means of checking the staff's scoring if the patient rates himself on a higher or lower score.

Sixteen staff (n = 21) have found it useful to incorporate the STAS assessment into the clinical setting and are using it as a method for evaluating their work and their patients.

This evaluation study does have recognized shortcomings. First, due to time constraint the questionnaires were only distributed to doctors and nurses in the palliative care and home care teams. The social worker, occupational therapist, chaplain and pastoral care worker were excluded from the sample. All members of the multi-professional team would provide information which would permit a more rigorous examination of the experience of the use of the STAS record. However, those respondents who participated in the study do provide a description of their experiences.

Second, there was a lengthy interval of ten months between introducing STAS and evaluating staff's experiences to its use. I would suggest that a three month evaluation time would be more appropriate. It is interesting to note that although audit is very popular, there is a dearth of information on the views of staff who take part in it. The evaluation described here was quick, easy and cheap to administer. I would recommend an anonymous questionnaire to others embarking on audit.

Clinical audit involves professionals working together in identifying objectives, defining standards, measuring performance and reviewing the results. We have now been using STAS for just over a year on a weekly basis. The ratings are agreed between all professionals at the team's weekly meetings and the observations are made within the normal course of care. Our next step is to analyse the results, to demonstrate areas of care which are most and least effective. We will use the Palliative Care Management System (PCMS), a personal computer data base incorporating STAS, to achieve this.

An important benefit of establishing audit in this way is that it systematizes thinking about the objectives and outcomes of care, thereby improving practice and completing the audit cycle. I would suggest that on reviewing all of the results, this system will be established as a permanent part of ward and home care practice.

References

1 Higginson I (1992) The development, validity, reliability and practicality of a new measure of palliative care—the Support Team Assessment Schedule. PhD thesis, University of London.

Further reading

Butters E, Higginson I, George R, Smith A and McCarthy M (1992) Assessing the symptoms, anxiety and practical needs of HIV/AIDS patients receiving palliative care. *Quality of Life Research* 1(1): 47–51.

Higginson I, Wade A and McCarthy M (1988) A comparison of four outcome measures of terminal care. In: Gilmore A, Gilmore S, (eds.), *A Safer Death: Multidisciplinary Aspects of Terminal Care*. New York, Plenum: 205–11.

Higginson I, Wade A and McCarthy M (1992) Effectiveness of two palliative support teams *Journal of Public Health Medicine* 14(1): 50–6.

Higginson I, Wade A and McCarthy M (1990) Palliative Care: Views of patients and their families. *British Medical Journal* 301: 277–81.

Higginson I and McCarthy M (1989) Evaluation of Palliative Care: Steps to quality assurance? *Palliative Medicine* 3: 267–74.

Higginson I and McCarthy M (1989) Measuring Symptoms in Terminal Cancer: Are pain and dyspnoea controlled? *Journal of the Royal Society of Medicine* 82:

Kitsun AL (1987) Raising Standards of Clinical Practice – The Fundamental Issue of Effective Nursing Practice. *Journal of Advanced Nursing* 12: 321–9.

Mayers MG (1972) A search for assessment criteria. *Nursing Outlook* 20(5): 323–6.

McCarthy M and Higginson I (1991) Clinical Audit by a Palliative Care Team. *Palliative Medicine* 5: 215–21.

Shaw CC and Costain DW (1989) Guidelines for Medical Audit: seven principles. *British Medical Journal* 299: 498–9.

16

Audit Experience: Views of a Hospice Director

ILORA FINLAY

Introduction

Medical audit was established in 1989 in our 38-bed palliative care centre (which also has home care and day care services). Within two years the process had evolved into clinical audit.

Methods

Acceptance of audit

Audit in our unit began with medical audit, partly because other disciplines were very reluctant to be involved[1]. Once the medical team were seen to be auditing their care on a regular basis, it became easier for other staff to join in the formalized process. However, the emotional difficulties for any of the team starting to appraise care should not be underestimated; it rapidly became evident that a few team members would use various avoidance tactics such as ensuring to be off duty at the date of the meeting or by being unable to leave the ward to attend the meeting.

Some ground rules (*see* Box 16.1) were established within the team for the audit meetings and proved effective at allaying these fears.

Audit in the team

Within the multidisciplinary team, there are small numbers of personnel other than nursing staff. The multidisciplinary nature of palliative care requires some blurring of roles but the individual responsibilities of each

> **Box 16.1:** Ground rules for audit
>
> 1. There is an ethical and moral obligation on all team members to audit their care.
> 2. All comments should be constructive; destructive criticisms should be avoided.
> 3. No matter how good our standard of care is, as perceived by ourselves, the patients and relatives, there is always room for improvement and updating.
> 4. The perception of the patient and their own carers should be considered as much as possible during the audit process, so that audit enhances patient-centred care.
> 5. Anonymized records of the meeting are kept and maintained in an open central file. It is the duty of all those present at the meetings to ensure that the findings are explained to as many members of staff as possible.
> 6. Clinical audit does not replace educational programmes; it is a source of education within the team.

discipline need to be clearly defined. Without clear role definition within the multidisciplinary team, there is an inherent danger of either too much responsibility being carried by one discipline, or conversely, for responsibilities from one discipline to be abdicated since they may appear to be being covered by another, eg in considering mouth care, nursing, medical, dietitian and dental services all have a role to play. It can be easy when inadequate care is highlighted for any one discipline to 'scapegoat' another; this must be avoided if clinical audit is to be constructive rather than destructive to the team.

The process

Case note review from randomly pulled case files was undertaken initially, but found to be non-productive. The meetings rapidly became 'self-congratulatory' where any aspect of care could be justified by whoever had been involved at the time. Within our unit, case review occurs at the regular clinical ward meetings where it is felt to be a useful and constructive process.

Topic audit[2] was therefore adopted whereby the audit cycle[3] could be easily implemented. The topic to be audited is decided by the audit meeting and then the minimum standards that we should be, or believe we are, achieving are defined (Phase I), based on the documented best current practice from literature[4] and as agreed by the group. Several qualitative aspects of palliative care are difficult to define with hard scientific data[5] so we feel consensus of opinion of the clinical audit group is particularly important when standards are set. After a minimum standard has been agreed, a selection of case notes are reviewed or a survey is undertaken (Phase II). This demonstrates whether the defined criteria are being met and identifies shortfalls in these standards. Then Phase III, to 'close the audit loop', is implemented. This involves deciding actions to be taken to rectify perceived deficit and then subsequently (Phase IV) re-evaluating to ascertain whether there is an improvement in reaching the standard target.

This is different from planning and evaluation by the nursing process, when the care plan is formulated on an individual basis and reviewed for the individual patient; in audit the standards set need to be applicable across the range of patients under the care of the unit.

The data base

The need for an accurate data base for audit from within the patient's clinical notes rapidly became evident. The first task of the group was to redesign the medical and nursing notes to ensure an adequate data base.

It was decided to evolve joint nursing and medical notes in which information could rapidly be identified regarding significant events in the patient's stay. A coding system for symptom evaluation with a 4-point scale was devised for each of 26 common symptoms. Each symptom is evaluated on a 0 (not present), 1 (mild), 2 (moderate), 3 (severe) scale. This rapid, although relatively crude, scoring of patient symptoms can be completed by the evaluating nurse on a regular basis and is held in the patient's notes (an example is shown in Figure 16.1). The aim is that this evaluation score is done in conjunction with the patient, although this has not yet been achieved. Nursing and medical notes are maintained in parallel in a chronological order within a grid system, so that problems can be seen at a glance (*see* Figure 16.2). All core sociodemographic data on the patient is recorded on an essential frontispiece which avoids duplication between nursing and medical notes.

Other paramedical staff (social work, physiotherapy and occupational therapy) also record in the single set of notes, which includes a referral form for bereavement follow-up of the carers.

The notes incorporate a communication sheet to record key conversations with patients or their carers, which is completed by whichever member of staff was involved in the key conversation and is cross-referenced onto the medical/nursing notes.

The acceptability of this new note format has been extremely high since the amount of writing to be undertaken by the nursing and medical

EVALUATION OF PROBLEMS   Score: 0-3/   0 = none;   1 = mild;
2 = moderate;   3 = severe

Problem	Admission								
1. Swallowing									
2. Anorexia									
3. Nausea									
4. Vomiting									
5. Urine									
6. Bowels									
7. Weight loss									
8. Oedema									
9. Dyspnoea									
10. Hearing									
11. Vision									
12. Speech									
13. Paresis									
14. Weakness									
15. Insomnia									
16. Confusion									
17. Fears/worries									
22. Self-care									
23. Pressure sores									
24. Mouth									
25. PAINS:									

Figure 16.1: Extract from patient notes

Continuation assessment

Nursing staff	Doctor
Date: AM .... PM .... Night	
Date: AM .... PM .... Night	
Date: AM .... PM .... Night	

Figure 16.2: Nursing and medical notes parallel grid system

staff has decreased. Obtaining information from the case notes has also become more efficient.

Data collection

Three ways of collecting data have been used (*see* Box 16.2).

Box 16.2: Data collection can be from:

1. Selection of notes for review (20 to 30 in total) are pulled at random by a member of the clerical staff. Randomization codes have not been used, although they could be useful to ensure a representative sample.
2. Census sampling has also been used to collect data, whereby all patients in the service (in-patients, day care patients and home care patients) on a particular day are surveyed as the source of data[6].
3. Patients known to have undergone a specific procedure are traced, eg for blood transfusion, the patient names were easily traced from blood bank records to give a total sample within a chosen time frame, such as two years. The computerization of the clinical data base on patients will assist with data collection on patients in this category.

Through these different methods, the sample size is between 40 and 100. This sampling is not restricted to in-patients, but includes day care and home care patients. The work in collecting data should not be underestimated. It is necessary to limit the sample size and clearly define the type of data to be obtained. This workload should be spread throughout the members of the group and should not be put onto the junior medical staff[7].

Topics we have looked at during our audit and the resulting changes in clinical practice

The following list describes the factors that we have looked at, and for each factor, the resulting changes in clinical practice.

1. Recording in case notes.
   - Case notes redesigned to multidisciplinary notes.
2. Drug chart errors.
   - Guidelines on completion of drug chart.

- Drug chart redesigned.
- Nurse initiated administration of certain proprietary medications from an agreed list.

3. Blood transfusion, shown in detail in the next section.

    - Guidelines evolved to give transfusion if patient is symptomatic from anaemia, likely to live more than two weeks and has low Hb (usually 8 Gms or less).

4. Random review of clinical decision making.

    - Process of random review abandonded in favour of topic audit in our pattern of work.

5. Restlessness in last days of life.

    - Use of midazolam increased.
    - Greater awareness of pain and need for frequent repositioning of patient unable to move.

6. Pressure sores.

    - Educational programme initiated for all staff. Beds reviewed. Turning schedules introduced. Holme Tower Risk Score evolved.

7. Factors affecting admission and discharge.

    - Admission procedures were supported by evidence from the audit. Our rapidly responsive service was justified, but staff skill mix was shown to be inadequate at times, resulting in revision of duty rotas. The evidence from the audit supported the implementation of team nursing.

8. Communication with GP whenever a patient dies or is discharged.

    - Notification to the GP adequately recorded on the case notes. A separate section was introduced in the case record where the nurse simply signed that the GP had been contacted and a clear directive issued.

9. Laxatives, fluid intake and constipation.

    - Identification of poor fluid intake amongst in-patients as a contributory factor to constipation when home care, day care and in-patients were compared.
    - Evolution of a laxative policy.
    - Volunteers brought in to undertake additional drinks rounds; ward routine reviewed to emphasize fluids and diet.

10.   Nausea and vomiting.

   ● Staff awareness of vomiting is good, but nausea alone tends
     to be underestimated by all staff. Anorexia as a pointer to
     nausea is often missed.

Example of one audit: indications for blood transfusion in palliative care

The audit cycle is shown in Figure 16.3.

Set objectives

Meeting 1: pre-audit phase 16 months
1.   State criteria: what we think we are using as transfusion criteria
     (pre-audit criteria).
2.   Trace patient's notes on all patients who have received transfusion
     over past 16 months via blood back records.
3.   Extract data from notes on:

   ● the reason for transfusion
   ● whether the patient benefited from transfusion or not
   ● the pre-transfusion Hb level.

4.   Discuss findings with consultant haematologist involved who was
     invited to attend the meeting.
5.   Redefine our transfusion criteria.
6.   Plan prospective data collection based on the new criteria (post-
     audit criteria).
7.   Fix date for follow-up meeting.

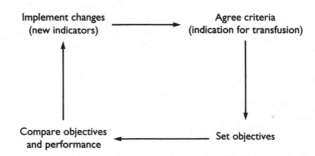

Figure 16.3: The audit cycle: indicators for blood transfusion

Compare objectives and performance

Meeting 2: follow up
Examine data collected during prospective post-audit phase.

- Question: Did more patients obtain symptomatic benefit from transfusion?
  Answer: Yes, especially relief of fatigue on minimal effort. $P < 0.1$.
- Question: Are our new criteria better for our patient care in terms of symptomatic improvement overall?
  Answer: Yes. $P < 0.1$.
- Question: Are patients only transfused when Hb < 8 Gms?
  Answer: No. Pre-audit 71% had Hb < 8 Gms before transfusion. Post-audit 73% had Hb < 8 Gms before transfusion.
- Question: Were any patients made symptomatically worse by transfusion?
  Answer: No

Implement changes

Meeting 3: conclusions
New criteria adopted which will result in slight increase in the use of blood transfusion in our patients. (Pre-audit 2.6% of patients transfused and post-audit 4.5% of patients transfused).

Compare objectives and performance

This is shown in Table 16.1.

Observe performance

Post-audit phase (five months). Log all patients transfused and assess benefits/adverse reactions to transfusion.

Symptom	Phase I – Pre-audit		Phase II – Post-audit	
	Number of patients:		Number of patients:	
	no benefit	benefit	no benefit	benefit
Fatigue	11	8	2	7
Dyspnoea	2	6	0	3
Postural hypotension	0	1	0	1
Bleeding	0	0	1	1
Total	13	15	3	12

Average number of units used per patient = 1.93 pre-audit, 2.47 post-audit.

Table 16.1: Comparison of objectives and performances: blood transfusion

---

Box 16.3: Indication for transfusion

Pre-audit	Post-audit
Transfusion considered if:	1. Haemoglobin < 8 Gms/dl
Haemoglobin < 8 Gms/dl *plus* Symptoms of anaemia *plus* Life expectancy > 6 weeks	Symptoms: ● dyspnoea ● fatigue on minimal exertion ● postural hypotension ● bleeding which may be stopped
2 units of packed cells given	2. If life expectancy > 2 weeks *plus* Symptoms Then transfuse if haemoglobin < 8 Gms/dl
= The criteria we thought we were using.	= The new criteria.

No post-transfusion Hb is indicated, since the blood is being given to obtain symptomatic improvement only.

Box 16.3 shows the new indications for transfusion.

Difficulties encountered

The implicit threat to perceived good care should not be under-estimated. Those feeling threatened can interpret audit initially as having some ulterior motive, or as providing a sleight on their standards of care. We have found that with reassurance and instruction by example these fears have rapidly resolved amongst the staff.

The timing of the meetings to allow maximum day and night senior staff attendance was initially difficult to determine; an 8.00 am meeting once a month has become adopted as the acceptable time. Meetings are limited to one hour in length so that the process of holding an audit meeting does not erode into patient care.

Recording the proceedings of the meeting is done by one of the staff present since it was felt inappropriate to have a secretary taking minutes. Because of the speed of writing and note taking, this function initially fell to the medical director, but has subsequently been taken on by the matron; it could be undertaken by any member of the meeting.

The chairperson of the meetings was chosen as a neutral member of the team. It is important that the chairperson is somebody widely trusted by all the staff. The chairperson must facilitate the concept of ownership rather than impose audit on staff. Individual staff must feel valued through the meetings. It is important for the chairperson to have a well-defined concept of audit and to be able to allow open discussion in which all present can participate without discussions becoming too heated; skill is sometimes required to avoid destructive criticism which would make team members feel undermined.

The cost implications

There are cost implications in establishing clinical audit. Staff time is taken in both preparation and attendance at audit meetings. Deficits identified require action taken which can have implications for capital expenditure, eg new record system, review of catering, and certainly for expenditure in terms of staff time to attain the necessary changes in clinical practice. Information technology, although useful, is not essential to the process of clinical audit in our current experience. However, a working knowledge of simple statistical techniques is extremely useful to be able to differentiate rapidly between significant differences in the sample size looked at and the occurrence of trends.

Closing the loop

There are difficulties in implementing change even when the changes are agreed at the meeting.
1. Cascading communication from those present at the meeting to the other staff does not occur adequately.
2. Those with hands-on patient contact, eg auxiliary nurses need to feel ownership of any changes, but they are often at the end of the cascade.
3. The main communicator may be a resistor to change. Many health care professionals have innate conservatism to resist change of long cherished views. This may be partly from fear of their deficits being revealed.

Continuing education is of paramount importance to achieve change. It is best targeted to ensure that those to be educated feel part of the teaching/learning process. One mechanism, which has shown some success, is by asking the full team of nurses to evolve the policy themselves, with the facilitation of the tutor.

Conclusion

It was anticipated that the defining of the topic for audit would be difficult. However, we have found that the ideas for topics to audit has far exceeded the speed with which we are able to tackle them and the list continues to evolve.

Attendance at meetings is hardest to obtain from those members of staff most reluctant to change their practices. However, audit has been a constructive medium through which to identify deficits in care and instigate changes. The process has been educative and the meetings stimulating and enjoyable. The chairperson is essential to maintain momentum and active cohesiveness of the group.

References

1 Bowden D and Walshe K (1991) When medical audit starts to count. *British Medical Journal* **303**: 101–3.

2 Royal College of Physicians (1989) *Medical audit: a first report*. London: RCP.

3 WHO Working Group (1989) The organisation of quality assurance. *Quality Assurance in Health Care* **1**: 111–23.

4 Bhopal RS and Thomson R (1991) A form to help learn and teach about assessing medical audit papers. *British Medical Journal* **303**: 1520–2.

5 Report of Working Group of the Research Unit of the Royal College of Physicians (1991) Palliative care: guidelines for good practice and audit measures. *Journal of Royal College of Physicians (London)* **25**(4): 325–8.

6 Fitzpatrick R (1991) Surveys of patient satisfaction: I – Important general considerations. *British Medical Journal* **302**: 887–9.

7 *Clinical audit in Wales* (1990) Welsh Council for Postgraduate Medical and Dental Education, 2; Part 1.

Further reading

Ford G (1990) Constructive audit. *Palliative Medicine* **4**(1): Editorial.

17

Audit Experience: Using a Data Base to Audit Care

ELIZABETH BUTTERS, IRENE HIGGINSON, FINBARR MURPHY AND
MAURA McDONNELL

Introduction

This chapter highlights some of the main considerations when developing, choosing and using personal computer data bases for audit. The Palliative Care Management System (PCMS), a personal computer data base incorporating the Support Team Assessment Schedule (STAS) (*see* Chapter 5) is used as an illustration of a computer-based audit system.

Why a personal computer data base?

There can be many advantages in using computer data bases (*see* Box 17.1). They can provide a quick, user-friendly way of collecting and analysing routine data and producing reports; thereby helping to close the feedback loop of the audit cycle.

However, computers have their limitations, they cannot do everything and they do not provide all the answers. Any information produced by a data base is only as accurate as the data which is entered and computers cannot set standards or effect change[1]. Box 17.2 lists some of their disadvantages.

Choosing and developing data bases

Any proposed audit must be well thought out and established before a computer data base is developed. Staff must be convinced of the value of the audit and trained in its use, so that they are committed to data collection, before a data base is introduced.

Box 17.1: Advantages of using computer data bases

- They give staff the ability to collect and analyse their own data.
- Data collection can be on-going and not limited by the confines of a special study or survey.
- Rapid access to data (ie patient details and audit data) is possible.
- They give staff the ability to carry out quick routine analysis of data.
- Data can be printed out and produced in various formats, which saves time. For example, patients' details, discharge and death summaries, lists of patients, statistics for reports, graphics and so on.
- Data can be transferred between different compatible data bases and packages. This allows data to be shared between different computer users, further analysis of data using statistical packages and the production of high quality print-out (ie graphics).
- The introduction of a computer data base gives staff the incentive and opportunity to acquire and update computing skills.

Box 17.2: Disadvantages of using computer data bases

- Staff may not have computer knowledge or skills and some may feel threatened by the introduction of a computer data base. Training in computer skills and the data base may take up valuable time.
- Additional resources may be necessary to buy, upgrade or run computers and data base packages can be expensive to buy and develop.
- The temptation is to try to get a data base to do everything, so it becomes very large and unwieldy.
- Potential additional workload and duplication of existing work. For example, if a computer print-out cannot be used as a substitute for handwritten notes.
- There is the risk of losing data. For example, if data is not saved after it has been entered or if the data base fails or is accidentally deleted. (NB An up-to-date back-up copy of the data base should always be available.)
- If the data base does not automatically back-up (make copies) of all data someone will have to take responsibility for this.
- Solving any problems or bugs which develop and modifying the data base may be expensive and time consuming.

Box 17.2: *Continued*

- There is a risk of unauthorized access to data, particularly if the data base works over a network or is on a mainframe compuer.
- There may be times when data cannot be accessed. For example, when shared personal computers are used.
- The data base may not be compatible with other computer data bases and packages.

The information which a computer data base produces is only as accurate as the data which is entered onto it. If staff do not understand how to correctly carry out the audit the information collected will be useless.

Data collection using a computer-based audit system should be part of normal working practice and staff should quickly be able to see the benefits of using the system.

The ideal way to obtain a data base which most exactly meets individual requirements is to develop one from scratch. However, this is a time consuming process (it took nearly two years to develop and test PCMS) and can be very expensive, so this is often not a feasible option. The best alternative is to choose and if necessary adapt an existing data base. Box 17.3 describes important considerations when choosing a data base.

Box 17.3: Things to consider when choosing a data base

- How much money is available to spend?
- Will it work with existing computer systems?
- Is it well known and reliable?
- Does it collect all the required data?
- Does it collect a large amount of data which is not required?
- How easy is it to modify?
- Does it carry out the necessary analysis of data?
- What print-outs are available (ie reports, graphics) and can new ones be created?
- Is it easy to learn and user-friendly?
- Does it include on-line help and easy to follow documentation (manuals)?
- Will it fit into normal working practice?
- What other features does it include (eg word processing) and how useful are they?
- How easy is it to transfer data to other data bases and packages (eg for further analysis or to produce high quality print-out)?

Any computer-based audit system (data base) whether it be developed from scratch or an existing data base must be:

- relatively cheap or give users value for money
- simple, easy to use and fit into normal working practice
- not include too much data or unreliable data
- flexible and easy to modify
- allow users to carry out routine analysis of data and to produce various print-out options
- reliable
- compatible with other software.

Single or multi-user systems?

A multi-user system (network version) allows the data to be used by more than one member of staff at a time, for example, staff working in different wards could enter data (at different computer terminals) at the same time, rather than having to take turns to use a single free-standing personal computer.

Avoid using mainframe computers although they do have some advantages; they can be expensive to use, users must learn operating systems which may change, there may be times when they are very slow and times when users cannot access them, and users may have to rely on computer staff for additional help and advice.

The Palliative Care Management System (PCMS)

Our aim in developing PCMS was to produce a cheap and user-friendly data base which would allow professionals providing palliative care to collect and analyse routine patient data and to audit their work.

PCMS incorporates existing validated audit measures: the Support Team Assessment Schedule (STAS) (*see* Chapter 5) and the Hebrew Rehabilitation Centre for Aged Quality of Life Index (HRCA-QL) – a modified version of Spitzer's Quality of Life Index[2,3]. Box 17.4 gives a summary of PCMS's main features. Box 17.5 shows an example of a patient record produced by PCMS.

How will data be entered?

It may take some time to train all staff to use a data base and often the secretary or administrator will be the only member of staff who has a computer and computer skills. Secretaries and administrators may be reluctant to take on the extra work of data entry if they see no direct benefit from it.

Box 17.4: Palliative Care Management System (PCMS)

PCMS includes the following features:

- Patients

Demographic, diagnostic and social detals of patients referred (*see* Box 17.5 and Box 17.6). Free fields allow users to record other relevant information. Free text notes can also be entered for each patient.

Existing codes have been used where possible eg for ethnic group (UK 1991 census codes) and diagnosis (International Classification of Disease codes).

- STAS (audit data)

Allows for routine (ie weekly/fortnightly) collection of audit data using STAS items (nine key fixed, seven optional items) and HRCA-QL items for HIV/AIDS patients. Users can select and define four additional audit items themselves. Suggestions are offered as to how items can be modified eg to audit individual symptoms or drugs.

Other information collected includes: place of care, contact information (ie UK Korner), details of discharge, re-admittance, death and initial bereavement follow up.

- Output

Allows patients' details to be printed out for use as notes (*see* Box 17.5). Graphs ratings of STAS items over time (*see* Figures 17.1 and 17.2). Lists of patients, address labels, discharge and death summaries, standard annual reports and statistics (ie UK Korner data for managers) can all be produced and printed out.

- Data validity checks, eg users are warned if dates are old or out of order.

- Help and documentation – lookup facilities: pull down menus of codes which can also be printed out. Comprehensive on-line help text which users can modify. Documentation (manuals) on disk. Notes about data base modifications.

- Security – passwords and security (access) levels. Exports numeric strings only.

- Advanced features – export and cleardown utilities:
  export allows users to transfer data to statistical packages for further analysis.
  Cleardown allows users to remove data (ie dead patients) from their data base.

- Modification – PCMS can easily be adapted for use by a variety of professionals providing palliative care to different patient groups in different settings.

Box 17.5: An example of a PCMS patient record

PCMS   Patient detailed record   Page 1

Name:	Joe Bloggs	Patient ID:	00001
Address:	66 Gower Road	Date created:	07/05/92
	London		
Postcode:	NW1 2RJ	'Phone – Home:	
		Work:	

Patient – Sex:	1 Male	District of residence:	9999 Missing
Marital status:	1 Married	Patient living with:	2 other people
Religion:	9 Missing	Accommodation:	1 owner occupied
Ethnic group:	0 White	Means of access:	1 ground floor
Date of birth:	01/04/29	Health cover:	0 NHS

Nearest carer:	1 Wife	Carer's Karnofsky	100 normal, no evidence of disease
Carer's work:	2 Full-time	Next of kin:	1 Wife
Carer name		Next of kin name	
and address:	Mary Bloggs	and address:	Same as carer
	66 Gower Road		
	London		
	NW1 2RJ		

Patient's GP (family doctor) name and address: 123 Dr J Smith
2 Briar Way
London
NW1 3PQ

'Phone:

Main diagnosis:	160 lung cancer	Other diagnosis (1):	725 rheumatism
Date of diagnosis:	04/91	Other diagnosis (2):	999 missing

Date of referral:	02/05/92	Other professionals (1):	2 district nurse
Patient referred by:	1 general practitioner	Other professionals (2):	99 missing
Name of referrer:	123 Dr J Smith	Medical card number:	99 missing
Place of care at referral:	1 home	Hospital number:	9999999999 missing
Reason for referral (1):	1 symptom control	Consultant name:	012 Dr P Jones
Reason for referral (2):	2 family anxiety	Speciality code:	015 radiotherapy

Remarks:

If clinical staff know how to use the data base (ie how to carry out data entry and analysis) they can have immediate access to patient and audit data, as well as the ability to produce their own reports.

If data must be entered in a standard way, for example, if the data base is case sensitive (ie upper/lower case), the less people who carry out the data entry the more accurate the data entry is likely to be.

Some clinical staff will choose to carry out their own data entry directly onto the computer data base; whereas others may dictate or hand write notes, which are later entered onto the data base by a secretary or administrator. If a secretary or administrator is carrying out the data entry it is important that they are given some incentive to carry out this additional work. Routine administrative tasks which could be carried out using a data base include word processing, producing letters, address labels, memos, summaries and so on, thus saving secretarial time elsewhere. However, additional features such as these increase the size of the data base.

The frequency of data collection and who actually carries out the data entry will be determined by a number of factors:

- patient group, eg cancer, HIV/AIDS, other
- setting, eg community (ie home, day care), in-patient (ie hospice, hospital)
- frequency and nature of contact with patients
- number of staff and resources (eg number and type of computers) available
- type of data collected.

Data to be included and collected

When deciding what data should be collected a number of factors need to be considered:

- **Who is the data being collected for?**

Service providers, management, funding bodies.

- **Is the information essential and how easy is it to collect?**

Do not try to include information on everything. The larger the data set the less likely it is that all the data will be collected and a lot of it may not be used or analysed – it will become 'orphan data'[4].

Do not include data which is difficult to collect. For example, there are many patient identification numbers which are not necessary or feasible to collect. Often neither the patient or professional will know what some of these numbers are and there is no point in trying to collect this information if it is not available. Keep the data set as minimal as possible, whilst ensuring that all essential information was included.

- **What audit measures should be included?**

There are a number of advantages to using existing validated audit measures: they save time, allow data collection to begin more quickly and allow for comparison with existing data.

- **How should data be coded?**

Developing new codes is a time consuming process and the use of existing codes means that the data collected will be compatible with data from other data sets.

Standardized codes should be fixed so that the user cannot change them. However, it is helpful if users can expand some of the existing code lists and are able to enter their own code lists for some items to take account of local circumstances. For example, the names of local referrers and GPs (family doctors) and codes used by their health district (management).

- **Data validity checks**

It is important that data is collected and entered correctly so that any information produced by the data base is valid and useful. Data validity checks for obvious errors should be included. For example, users can be warned if dates are out of order (ie date of death or discharge is before date of referral). Print-out of patient details and audit data can also be used to see if data has been entered correctly.

Data base modifications

It is impossible to foresee changing information requirements so any computer-based audit system must be easy for the user to modify.

The inclusion of user-defined fields allows for variations in users requirements and for the collection of additional data in the future. It is helpful if some suggestions as to ways in which users can modify the data base are provided.

Some documentation or help about data base modifications for both users and more experienced computer programmers, who may wish to make more extensive alterations to the data base, should be provided.

Use well known and readily available software.

Analysis

If a data base is to be useful it must allow the user to carry out some routine, basic analysis of data collected, whether it analyses the data itself or puts it into a format which can be transferred into another computer package for analysis. Data analysis should not be too complicated.

Output – print-out

Data bases should provide useful, reasonable quality print-out, which can often save secretarial time, for example by producing patient notes and summaries, preparing reports and graphics.

It is important that the print-out from a data base is in a format which its users like and will use. (*See* Figures 17.1 and 17.2 for examples of graphics produced by PCMS.)

Report building packages are available which allow users to develop their own print-out formats.

Use well known and readily available printer options.

Ease of use (user-friendliness)

There is no point in having a data base which users find hard to understand and use. Where possible on-screen command menus and pull down code lists should be provided, as well as access to on-screen help text and easy to follow documentation (manuals). It is also helpful if the user can print out code lists and modify the help text.

There are a number of advantages to producing documentation (manuals) on disk: documentation can be viewed on screen, it reduces the overall cost of the data base, saves paper and postage costs, and allows users to produce multiple copies of the documentation.

Data confidentiality and security

The data base should be password protected. Different operator codes and access levels for different users can also be used. For example, high access levels to allow users to make extensive modifications to the data base, whilst lower access levels can be given to less experienced users who only carry out routine data entry and analysis, so that there is no danger that the data base will be altered or damaged by less experienced users.

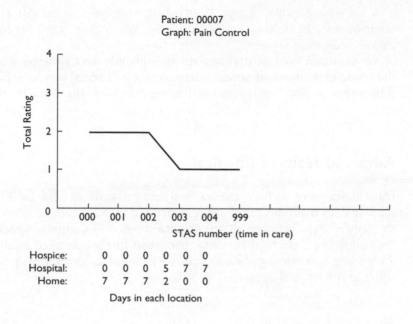

Figure 17.1: Graphic output from PCMS: an individual patient's ratings for pain control during the course of their care

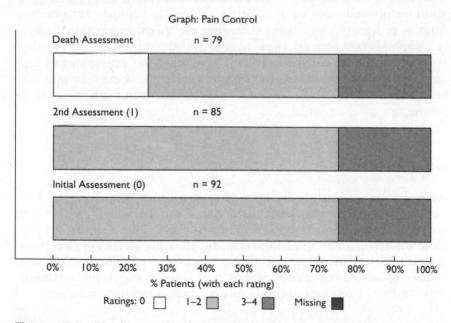

Figure 17.2: Graphic output from PCMS: the percentage of patients with different ratings for pain control at different points in care

A log of use, which keeps a record of who has carried out actions, what actions have been carried out and when they were taken, is a useful additional feature.

To maintain confidentiality data should only be exported from the data base in the form of numeric strings (*see* Advanced features, below). Remember to find out if you need to register with the Data Protection Act.

Advanced features (utilities)

Data bases may include export and import utilities and facilities to remove data from the data base. Export and import utilities allow users to transfer data between different data bases and computer packages, thus allowing them to share data, carry out further detailed analysis of data using statistical packages and to produce high quality print-out using graphics packages.

Testing the data base

Whilst developing, testing and piloting a data base, seek the advice of a variety of people. Some time should be allowed to carry out a pilot study before full scale data collection begins. It is important that any bugs or problems which users encounter are sorted out at this stage. It is also important to seek users' opinions of the data base, before they commit their data collection to it. Users may, for example, feel that some important information or features have been omitted, or that help text and documentation are not comprehensive enough or easy to follow.

Conclusions

An audit method must be well thought out before a computer data base can be developed. Computer data bases can be useful in the data collection and analysis stages of the audit cycle. They can also help to close the feedback loop of the cycle, by allowing staff rapid access to information about patients and the processes and outcome of care. However, computers have their limitations, they cannot do everything. Any statistics produced are only as accurate as the data entered.

References

1 Crombie I and Davies H (1991) Computers in audit: servants or sirens? *British Medical Journal* **303**: 403–4.

2 Morris J, Suissa S, Sherwood S, Wright S and Greer D (1986) Last days: a study of the quality of life of terminally ill cancer patients. *Journal of Chronic Diseases* **39**(1): 47–62.

3 Morris J and Sherwood S (1987) Quality of life in cancer patients at different stages in their disease trajectory. *Journal of Chronic Disease* **40**: 545–53.

4 Crombie and Davies, Computers in audit, *BMJ* **303**: 403–4.

Further reading

Department of Health (1990) *Medical audit: guidance for hospital clinicians on the use of computers*. London: HMSO.

Ellis B (1989) How to set up an audit. *British Medical Journal* **298**: 1635–7.

Rigby M, McBride A and Shiels C (1992) *Computers in medical audit: a guide commissioned by the West Midlands Regional Health Authority*. London: Royal Society of Medical Services.

Shaw C (1989) *Medical audit a hospital handbook*. (2nd edition) London: King's Fund Centre.

Smith A (1992) How to do it: design a clinical information system. *British Medical Journal* **305**: 415–17.

Tyndal R, Kennedy S, Naylop S, Pajak F, Lattimer W and Edwards N (1990) *Computers in medical audit*. London: Royal Society of Medicine.

18

Clinical Audit in Palliative Care:
A Critical Appraisal

ANTHONY HOPKINS

This chapter aims to pull together some of the themes covered elsewhere in the book. To these I have added some observations of my own. I have never worked in a hospice, but for a number of years I have been interested in evaluating the effectiveness of medical interventions, and, more recently, in evaluating the quality of medical care. My perspective therefore, is that of a 'friendly observer' outside palliative care, informed by helping organize a workshop on good practice in the field[1].

Multidisciplinary care

The first theme that runs through many of the chapters is the need for audit of palliative care to be multidisciplinary in nature. As Shaw outlines in Chapter 1, quality assurance in the 1980s tended to be led by the nursing profession, as many of the directors of quality assurance appointed in response to the Griffith's report on management came from the nursing profession[2]. The Royal College of Physicians set up a Working Party on Medical Audit in 1987, which reported in 1989[3], and the white paper *Working for Patients* was published in the same year[4]. These last two documents obviously centred upon the interventions of the medical profession, but within a short time it became apparent that medical audit could not be dissociated from the total package of care delivered by all members of the clinical care team. For example, it would be hopeless to audit the management of patients with stroke without involving the contributions of nurses, physiotherapists and occupational therapists. Indeed, medical interventions in the management of stroke are remarkably few.

Palliative care, by its very nature, is more multidisciplinary than most. Nurses, GPs, hospital consultants in a variety of specialties, social workers and chaplains or workers in other religions all play a part in making easier the passage to death. The Department of Health now clearly recognizes that audit is multidisciplinary in nature, the chief medical officer and chief nursing officer jointly chairing a new Clinical Outcomes Group, which is the primary Departmental vehicle for considering aspects of audit of the quality of care provided to patients. All writers of chapters in this book recognize the multidisciplinary nature of what is now commonly referred to as clinical audit.

Ethical considerations

The next theme I wish to discuss is the question of the ethics of clinical audit. For example, in a first draft of Chapter 9 sent to me by the editor, Bruera wrote that the cognitive function of the patients in his study was assessed using the Folstein Mini Mental State Questionnaire[5] *after informed consent was obtained*. The Folstein questionnaire is a brief questionnaire of ten items including such non-contentious questions as what day of the week it is. It seems to me an entirely proper function of a nurse or doctor to assess the cognitive function of his or her patient, as this reflects the way in which care is subsequently provided. Not to recognize that a patient's cognitive ability was impaired would be poor practice; furthermore, if the patient was severely cognitively impaired, he or she would not be able to give informed consent. I would argue that ethical committees should not require informed consent for assessments which are part of good clinical practice. The ethics of approaching bereaved relatives are considered, quite properly, in more detail by Addington-Hall and McCarthy in Chapter 10, and this is clearly an area where views may differ. This is reflected in the authors' observation that 'some committees were satisfied that the studies presented no major ethical problems and that the proposed study design took adequate account of both the need to be sensitive to bereaved relatives and the need to ensure informed consent was obtained, others expressed considerable alarm at the idea of intruding on the grief of bereaved people.' Where bodies of responsible people serving on different ethical committees can take diametrically opposed views, it is clear that there is no right or wrong answer. The view I would take is that it is ethically wrong to continue a type of professional practice the effectiveness of which has not been evaluated.

Clinical research versus clinical audit

Here we touch on the difference between clinical research and audit. In general, clinical research is a focused piece of work on a defined population in order to discover what ought to be done to improve health outcomes. Clinical audit determines whether what ought to be done (as discovered by research) is being done in the care setting which is being audited. In this particular example, clinical research might determine whether the relatives of deceased patients were better supported by one intervention than another. If the research showed a clear benefit for one intervention, then all that clinical audit would need to do subsequently would be to ensure that such intervention was being regularly undertaken, in preference to the less successful intervention. It would not be necessary to interview the bereaved relatives each time, as research would have already shown the benefits of the first intervention. However, local variations in the characteristics of patients and in the socio-economic and cultural characteristics of bereaved relatives might well mean that the benefits of research could not be readily transposed to another care setting. Even for this example, therefore, a small piece of local true research may be necessary.

The differences of opinion expressed by different local research ethics committees of which the example shown on page 169 is illustrative, has led to the suggestion from a number of quarters that there ought to be some sort of national ethics committee, in order to give guidance about research and audit in areas where there are genuine differences of opinion. For example, a hospice may receive patients from within the boundaries of four or five different health authorities; it would be very difficult if ethical permission were given for the interview of some relatives but not for others.

On a different ethical point, some colleagues are concerned about who has the right of access to medical and nursing and similar records for the purposes of clinical audit. The Audit Working Group of the Conference of Medical Royal Colleges and their faculties in the United Kingdom has recently published some guidelines on this topic[6].

There are, however, some similarities between research and clinical audit which do require consideration. Most important of all is the need for some proven methodology, an aspect addressed by a number of chapter authors, notably by the editor in Chapter 3. For example, Higginson points out that if severely ill patients cannot be assessed by interview, then the results obtained from the interview sample will be biased, and will not necessarily reflect the population as a whole of those being audited.

Special needs

It would also be a mistake to assume that the population of patients in hospices is homogeneous. In Chapter 11, Butters et al. show that there are distinct differences between patients with HIV/AIDS and cancer patients which need to be considered. Box 11.2 in their chapter shows that patients with HIV/AIDS tend to be younger, have more complex networks of carers, and a wider variety of medical presentations and problems requiring more complicated management. They are also less involved with their GPs. This means that audit of the care of these patients needs to address a number of problems that do not arise in patients with cancer. Equally common, from my own experience as a neurologist with patients with motor neurone disease, are specific problems relating to communication due to anarthria, swallowing and nutrition and immobility that may require quite a different range of support from that required by patients terminally ill with different forms of cancer. The important message here, I believe, is to recognize that an assessment schedule derived from interviews from patients, their carers and from experienced professional staff may not be thoughtlessly used for the assessment of patients with quite different characteristics. The work in this volume is, I believe, along exactly the right lines, in attempting to define the special needs of patients with different characteristics, and to develop methods to determine whether those needs are met.

However carefully an assessment schedule is developed, people are only terminally ill once, and they will have very ill-formed expectations both of the process of dying, and also of the likely success of the interventions that are possible. Such ill-formed expectations may not be easily captured by a schedule. Furthermore, their individual concerns will be individual by definition. One woman may be concerned by the financial problems that she is leaving behind, and another overwhelmingly concerned by pain or breathlessness.

Communication and the individuality of the patient

The two great criticisms of medical practice that patients consistently make is first, the failure of communication, which is, I believe, adequately recognized in all the chapters, and secondly the routinization of their individual problems. To take an example from my own speciality, a neurologist examining a patient who comes in complaining of a weak hand and who sees that the hand is wasted, will immediately start thinking 'I wonder if this is an ulnar nerve palsy; I wonder if this is motor neurone disease; I wonder if this is a cervical radicular lesion?' His questioning will be immediately focused along these lines, although the patient may be far more interested in saying how he has difficulty in opening the front door of his house since his hand has become weak, a matter of only anecdotal and trivial interest to the neurologist. The point about this digression is to indicate that there is some danger that formal assessment schedules, by attempting to fit the concerns of the patients into boxes on a proforma or into fields on a computer data base

(Chapter 17) may mean that the patients' individual concerns fail to be recognized as such and adequately addressed. A hint that this may be happening comes from Chapter 15, in which Table 15.4 shows that 10 out of 21 in-patient and home care staff members felt that the Support Team Assessment Schedule (STAS) failed to show a clear picture of the patient. When it is remembered that a third of the same respondents in this study from Dublin remarked that a schedule increased the work-load, and that the author of the STAS herself in Chapter 5 (*see* page 44) remarks that all care teams would have liked fewer items, here are warnings that a schedule is only one of a number of possible answers for clinical audit. A further indicator of the relative insensitivity of clinical assessment was shown in the validation of the Edmonton Symptom Assessment System, Chapter 8. Nurses were poor at assessing the overall sense of well-being described by patients, and although physicians showed a better correlation with the patient's own assessment on admission, again there was no correlation after the first few days[7].

Although schedules may be useful in helping patients and experienced staff identify goals, which, if achieved, become outcomes of the inter-ventions of palliative care, another approach may be to ask the in-dividual patient to define and the staff to record, say, three goals, which, if achieved, would reflect good individualized care. I ack-nowledge that this is in many ways a rather unreal statement. First of all, severely ill patients may be so frightened, confused and uncertain that they are unable to think exactly what they do want. Second, some goals which they would like to achieve may clearly not be achievable, for example, the correction of the financial problems that they are leaving behind. Third, goals and their priorities may change rapidly. Nonetheless, the point that I would like to keep right in the front of our minds is that no audit schedule, however good, will sufficiently address individual patient needs.

Members of the palliative care team must avoid the trap into which acute hospital staff have fallen for so many years – acquiring informa-tion because it is easily measured, (eg respiration rates) even though the data do not determine the outcomes of patient care.

Another related *caveat* is the managerial jargon that may indicate a mind-set that is not conducive to individualized patient care. Here I am thinking of the words 'officer', 'facilitator', 'baseline awareness', 'steering group', 'standardized auditing', all of which figure in a few lines of Chapter 9 on page 86. Overwhelmingly, palliative care is humane and individual, and although obviously it must be delivered within organized structures, it seems to me that these should, as far as possible, be concealed from the patient.

On the positive side, assessment schedules may be useful at picking up patient problems that would have gone unnoticed by an inex-perienced assessor, by reminding them of appropriate areas in which questions should be asked. They may also show the relative insufficiency of our present methods for relieving some symptoms, notably dyspnoea, as shown in Chapter 5, Figure 5.5. This is an example where clinical audit has shown up a need for further research.

Conclusion

My colleagues writing before me in this book have clearly shown that audit of palliative care has as its focus of interest appropriate outcomes which are specific to palliative care and distinct from care provided by those of us working in acute hospitals. Colleagues stress the multidisciplinary nature of the work, the need to encompass the family as well as the individual patient, and the need to pay particular attention to the timeliness of palliative care – when it is appropriate to start, and the need to continue after death by support of the bereaved relatives. As well as ensuring that good systems of audit are in place for patients in their care, those working in the specialty should ensure that their care is available to all sections of the community, including ethnic minorities[1,8] and the poor[9].

Acknowledgements

The Research Unit of the Royal College of Physicians is supported by generous grants from the Wolfson and Welton Foundations, by other charitable donations, and by the Department of Health.

References

1 Working Group of the Research Unit of the Royal College of Physicians (1991) Guidelines for good practice in palliative medicine. *Journal of the Royal College of Physicians of London* 25: 325–8.

2 Department of Health and Social Security (1983) *National Health Service Management Enquiry*. London: HMSO.

3 Royal College of Physicians (1989) *Medical audit – a first report*. London: Royal College of Physicians.

4 Department of Health (1989) *Working for patients*. Working Paper 6. London: HMSO.

5 Folstein MF, Folstein SE and McHugh PR (1975) Mini Mental State: A practical method for grading the cognitive state of patients for the clinician. *Journal of Psychiatric Research* 12: 189–98.

6 Audit Working Group of the Conference of Medical Royal Colleges and their Faculties in the United Kingdom (1992) Access to medical records for the purposes of medical audit. *British Medical Journal* **306:** 912.

7 MacEachern E (1992) *A study to determine the reliability and validity of the Edmonton Symptom Assessment System (ESAS).* Abstract. Presented at the 9th International Congress on the care of the terminally ill, Montreal, Canada, October 31–November 4.

8 Hopkins A and Bahl V (eds) (1993) *Access to health care for people from black and ethnic minorities.* London: Royal College of Physicians.

9 Cartwright A (1992) Social class differences in health and care in the year before death. *Journal of Epidemiology and Community Health* **46:** 54–7.

Appendix A: Support Team Assessment Schedule: Definitions and Ratings

General points

- The problem and need for improvement is scored on a five-point (0 to 4) scale at first contact, then weekly until death.
- High scores indicate many problems, low scores few problems.
- Family = the patient's nearest carer (ie parent, partner, relative or friend). *NB* This may change over time.
- Other professionals = the other involved professionals including GP, district nurse, social worker, hospital staff.
- Record 9 if you are unable to assess an item to indicate a missing score.
- Record 8 if the item is not applicable. (For example, when scoring family anxiety and insight if there is no carer.) This indicates a different missing score.
- Record 7 for all items for weeks when there was no contact with the patient or family.

Note on calculating total scores

- You cannot calculate a total score if you have any missing items (ie scores of 7 or 9). (If necessary you can extrapolate back from scores once they are known. For example, if the score of family insight is not known in the first week, but known to be 2 in the second week then you could assume it was also 2 in the first week.)
- If you have recorded an 8 (not applicable) then you can assume this is 0, if it is not applicable (eg no family) throughout care.

- For further information please contact:
  Dr Irene Higginson
  Senior Lecturer/Consultant
  Health Services Research Unit
  London School of Hygiene and Tropical Medicine
  Keppel Street
  London WC1E 7HT
  UK.

You are free to use the Support Team Assessment Schedule (STAS), but if you do intend to use it or an adapted version, place let us know in writing and acknowledge us in any written material or presentations.

Core (Higginson) nine items — to be assessed for all patients

Pain control
Effects of his/her pain on the patient.

0 = None.
1 = Occasional or grumbling single pain. Patient is not bothered to be rid of symptom.
2 = Moderate distress, occasional bad days, pain limits some activity possible within extent of disease.
3 = Severe pain present often. Activities and concentration markedly affected by pain.
4 = Severe and continuous overwhelming pain. Unable to think of other matters.

Other symptom control
Effects of his/her symptoms on the patient (not including pain).

0 = None.
1 = Occasional or grumbling single or few symptom(s). Patient has usual activity and is not bothered to be rid of symptom.
2 = Moderate distress, occasional bad days, symptoms limit some activity possible within extent of disease.
3 = Severe symptom(s) present often. Activities and concentration markedly affected by symptom(s).
4 = Severe and continuous overwhelming symptom(s). Unable to think of other matters.

Patient anxiety
Effects of his/her anxiety on the patient.
0 = None.

1 = Worry over changes. No physical or behavioural symptoms of anxiety. Concentration not affected.
2 = Waiting for changes or problems: on edge. Occasional physical or behavioural symptoms of anxiety.
3 = Anxious often. Physical/behavioural symptoms. Concentration markedly affected.
4 = Completely and continuously preoccupied with anxiety and worries. Unable to think of other matters.

Family anxiety
Effects of anxiety on the family.

Family = patient's nearest carer(s). Please specify who in the comments section, eg parents, relatives, partner, friends. *NB* This may change over time. Please note changes in the comments section.

0 = None.
1 = Worry over changes. No physical or behavioural symptoms of anxiety. Concentration not affected.
2 = Waiting for changes or problems: on edge. Occasional physical or behavioural symptoms of anxiety.
3 = Anxious often. Physical/behavioural symptoms. Concentration markedly affected.
4 = Completely and continuously preoccupied with anxiety and worries. Unable to think of other matters.

Patient insight
Patient's awareness of his/her prognosis.

0 = Full awareness of prognosis.
1 = Prognosis over or underestimated by up to 200%. For example, thinking the prognosis is six months when it is likely to be two to three.
2 = Uncertain over becoming well or long prognosis. For example 'Some people with this die and I might too soon'.
3 = Unrealistic. For example, expecting to return to normal activity or work for a year when the prognosis is only three months.
4 = Expecting to become completely well.

Family insight
Family's awareness of the prognosis.

0 = Full awareness of prognosis.
1 = Prognosis over or underestimated by up to 200%. For example, thinking the prognosis is six months when it is likely to be two to three.
2 = Uncertain over patient becoming well or long prognosis. For example 'Some people with this die and he/she might too'.

3 = Unrealistic. For example, expecting to return to normal activity or work for a year when the time scale is only three months.
4 = Expecting the patient to become completely well.

Communication between patient and family
Depth and openness of communication between patient and family.

0 = Communicating openly and honestly. Verbally and non verbally.
1 = Communicating openly at some times or with some family members, or sometimes with partner or with some members of family.
2 = Acknowledge condition but discussion does not satisfy either the patient or family who feel full implications are not discussed, or maybe with partner but not family.
3 = Out of step, all discussions guarded.
4 = Pretending.

Communication between professionals
Speed, accuracy and depth of information communicated between other professionals, reflecting any difficulties for patient and family. (Comment on who is involved.)

0 = Detailed correct messages to all involved on the same day.
1 = Correct messages between key professionals, minor inaccuracies and delays between others.
2 = Small changes in management not communicated/major changes delayed for over one day, between key professionals.
3 = Delay of several days to one week before major changes notified. For example, hospital to GP.
4 = Prolonged delays or no communication, professionals unsure of which other professionals are visiting and when.

Communication from professionals to patient and family
Depth of information given to patient and family, when they require this, from other professionals.

0 = Full information. Patient and family feel free to ask.
1 = Information communicated but not clearly understood.
2 = Facts given on request, patient or family would have liked more information.
3 = Evasive, avoids true picture or some questions.
4 = Avoids answering questions or visiting/gives incorrect information which distresses patient and family.

Additional items

Planning

Further need for the patient, as desired, to organize his/her affairs and special meetings. (This can be scored for the team in some cases, eg if the patient is demented. A note should be made of this in the comments section as above.)

0 = Completed or unnecessary.
1 = One aspect needs planning, not urgent, may be already underway.
2 = One aspect needs planning urgently/several aspects with some time available, may have been discussed.
3 = Major decisions to be made, urgent, patient has time to contribute and may have begun to think of these.
4 = Major decisions outstanding, muddled, very little time or capacity to plan or make arrangements. For example, deterioration or death imminent.

Practical aid

Further need for practical aids at home, reflecting the difficulty for patient and family without aids.

0 = None needed.
1 = One aid desirable, not urgent, patient managing present.
2 = One aid needed urgently ie the next day, or a few aids needed soon, patient or family experiencing some difficulty.
3 = Aids needed badly, some improvisation possible.
4 = Patient incapacitated without basic aids.

Financial

Further need for entitled benefits, reflecting the difficulty for patient and family without benefits. Benefits/grants from voluntary organizations are also included here.

0 = All entitled benefits received, managing.
1 = One benefit desirable, patient and family managing, matter may be in hand.
2 = One benefit required urgently/several benefits desirable, patient and family experiencing difficulties in managing.
3 = Urgent need for several benefits, barely managing.
4 = Not managing, entitled to many benefits, in chaos and none in hand.

Wasted time
Amount of patient's time lost for tests or appointments which could have been avoided, the patient not wishing to attend.

0 = No time lost.
1 = One to three hours lost. For example, trip for prescription which tired patient.
2 = Half to one day wasted. For example, out-patient appointment.
3 = One plus day wasted.
4 = Two plus days wasted. For example, unnecessary or prolonged admission, results lost and repeated etc.

Spiritual
Degree to which the patient is content with their own spiritual beliefs or philosophy.

0 = Content in self and world view, without feelings of guilt or punishment over illness. Any denomination or agnostic.
1 = Occasional doubts or unrealistic expectations. Patient able to resolve their feelings/problems themselves.
2 = Uncertain, sometimes troubled. Doubts. Patient unable to resolve their feelings/problems themselves.
3 = Uncertain and guilty. For example, troubled, conflicts, worry.
4 = Distraught with uncertainty or guilt over beliefs. In chaos as to how to remedy situation. Crisis, unable to resolve things, inability to cope, symptomatic (physical/emotional).

Professional anxiety
Effects of anxiety on other professionals reflecting any difficulties this causes for patient and family.

0 = None.
1 = One professional anxious. No inappropriate action.
2 = One or more professional(s) anxious, beginning to lose objectivity.
3 = Professional(s) stressed, multiple telephone calls, inappropriate action.
4 = Multiple indiscriminate referrals/want patient taken over/total paralysis.

Advising professionals
Amount and speed of advice needed for other professionals.

0 = No further advice needed.
1 = One professional needs advising within one week.
2 = One professional needs advising in one to two days/two plus professionals need advising within one week.

3 = Urgent/immediate advice needed for several professionals.
4 = Major difficulties of patient and family not recognized by key professionals.

Extra item sometimes used

Team anxiety
Effects of anxiety on the team reflecting any difficulties this causes for patient and family.

0 = None.
1 = One professional anxious. No inappropriate action.
2 = One or more professional(s) anxious, beginning to lose objectivity.
3 = Professional(s) stressed, multiple telephone calls, inappropriate action.
4 = Multiple indiscriminate referrals/want patient taken over/total paralysis.

Appendix B Definitions and Ratings for Individual's Symptoms which can be Added to STAS

(*see* Chapter 14)

Lymphoedema
Effects of his/her oedema on the patient.

0 = None.
1 = Slight oedema. Has usual activity and is not bothered to be rid of oedema.
2 = Moderate oedema – occasional bad days – symptoms limit some activity, for example legs feel heavy when walking.
3 = Severe oedema, activities and concentration markedly affected because of it.
4 = Severe and overwhelming oedema. Unable to think of other matters.

Dyspnoea
Effects of his/her dyspnoea on the patient.

0 = None.
1 = Occasional dyspnoea. Has usual activity and is not bothered to be rid of dyspnoea.
2 = Moderate dyspnoea, occasional bad days; dyspnoea limits some activity possible within extent of disease.
3 = Severe dyspnoea, present often. Activities and concentration markedly affected by dyspnoea.
4 = Severe and continuous overwhelming dyspnoea. Unable to think of other matters.

Anorexia
Effects of his/her anorexia on the patient.

0 = None.
1 = Occasional or grumbling anorexia. Has usual activity and is not bothered to be rid of anorexia.
2 = Moderate distress from anorexia, occasional bad days, anorexia limits some activity possible within extent of disease.
3 = Severe distress from anorexia present often. Activities and concentration markedly affected by anorexia.
4 = Severe and continuous overwhelming distress from anorexia. Unable to think of other matters.

Nausea
Effects of his/her nausea on the patient.

0 = None.
1 = Occasional nausea. Has usual activity and is not bothered to be rid of nausea.
2 = Moderate nausea, occasional bad days; nausea limits some activity possible within extent of disease.
3 = Severe nausea, present often. Activities and concentration markedly affected by nausea.
4 = Severe and continuous nausea. Unable to think of other matters.

Pressure areas/skin
This is an assessment of the distress to the patient because of skin/pressure area discomfort.

0 = None.
1 = Occasional or slight discomfort. Has usual activity and is not bothered to be rid of symptoms.
2 = Moderate discomfort: occasional bad days because of skin/pressure area discomfort, some activities limited.
3 = Severe discomfort, activities and concentration markedly affected.
4 = Severe and continuous discomfort. Unable to think of other matters.

Pruritus
Effects of his/her pruritus on the patient.

0 = None.
1 = Occasional or slight itch. Has usual activity and is not bothered to be rid of itch.

2 = Moderate distress from itch, occasional bad days. Itch limits some activity.

3 = Severe distress from itch, present often. Activities and concentration markedly affected.

4 = Severe and continuous itch. Unable to think of other matters.

Constipation
Effects of his/her constipation on the patient.

0 = None.

1 = Occasional or grumbling constipation. Has usual activity and is not bothered to be rid of constipation.

2 = Moderate constipation, occasional bad days because of bowels.

3 = Severe constipation – present often. Activities and concentration markedly affected by bowel habit.

4 = Severe and overwhelming constipation. Unable to think of other matters.

Diarrhoea
Effects of his/her diarrhoea on the patient.

0 = None.

1 = Occasional or slight diarrhoea. Has usual activity and is not bothered to be rid of diarrhoea.

2 = Moderate diarrhoea, occasional bad days: diarrhoea limits some activity possible within extent of disease.

3 = Severe diarrhoea – present often. Activities and concentration markedly affected by diarrhoea.

4 = Severe and overwhelming diarrhoea. Unable to think of other matters.

Cough
Effects of his/her cough on the patient.

0 = None.

1 = Occasional or slight cough. Has usual activity and is not bothered to be rid of cough.

2 = Moderate cough with occasional bad days. Cough limits some activity.

3 = Severe cough present often. Activities (eg sleep) and concentration markedly affected by cough.

4 = Severe and continuous cough. Unable to think of other matters.

Haemoptysis – present Yes/No

Dysphagia

Remember – scoring is assessment of patient's distress from this symptom not necessarily severity of dysphagia itself.

0 = None.
1 = Occasional or slight dysphagia. Has usual activity and is not bothered to be rid of dysphagia.
2 = Moderate distress from dysphagia, occasional bad days: dysphagia limits some activity possible within extent of disease eg refusing food when offered if out visiting.
3 = Severe distress from dysphagia – present often. Activities and concentration markedly affected by dysphagia.
4 = Severe and continuous distress from dysphagia. Unable to think of other matters – it may mean patient unable to swallow anything and distressed by this.

Vomiting

Effects of his/her vomiting on the patient.

0 = None.
1 = Occasional or slight vomiting. Has usual activity and is not bothered to be rid of vomiting.
2 = Moderate amount of vomiting, occasional bad days – vomiting limits some activity possible within extent of disease (eg will not go out in case he/she is sick).
3 = Severe vomiting present often: activities and concentration markedly affected by vomiting.
4 = Severe and continuous vomiting. Unable to think of other matters.

Oral discomfort

This is to assess the degree of distress to the patient eg dry mouth may be a problem but a coated tongue may not. Would also include sore tongue, ill-fitting dentures (if annoying to patient). Does not include dysphagia.

0 = None.
1 = Occasional or grumbling oral discomfort. Has usual activity and is not bothered to be rid of oral problem.
2 = Moderate oral discomfort, occasional bad days, discomfort limits some activity possible within extent of disease eg not wearing dentures because of sore gums.

3 = Severe oral discomfort – present often. Activities and concentration markedly affected by oral discomfort.
4 = Severe and continuous oral discomfort. Unable to think of other matters.

Appendix C: Four New Items Developed by Our Lady's Hospice

(*see* Chapter 15)

Patient well-being (patient perspective) (provisional scoring)
Does the patient feel that he/she is doing okay in him/herself?

0 = Yes.
1 = Mostly yes.
2 = Yes and no.
3 = Mostly no.
4 = No.

Patient well-being (staff perspective) (provisional scoring)
Do we as a team feel that the person is doing okay in him/herself?

0 = Yes.
1 = Mostly yes.
2 = Yes and no.
3 = Mostly no.
4 = No.

Family well-being (provisional scoring)
Do we as a team feel that this family are doing okay in themselves?

0 = Yes.
1 = Mostly yes.
2 = Yes and no.
3 = Mostly no.
4 = No.

Staff anxiety (provisional scoring)
Effect of anxiety on professional caring for the patient/family?

0 = Happy.
1 = Mostly happy.
2 = Yes and no.
3 = Mostly unhappy.
4 = Unhappy.

NB These scorings have not been tested for reliability.

Appendix D: Draft Form for Use when Auditing Case Notes

(*see* Chapter 7)

Unit consultant: .... Date: ....

Auditor: ....

> Patient's name and details are NOT to be included
> in order to maintain strict confidentiality

	YES	NO	N/A not apply	INAD inadequate
DIAGNOSIS:				
A. DETAILS OF ADMISSION				
i Is the source of referral documented?				
ii Is the initial referral information adequate?				
iii Are the reasons for admission documented?				
iv Do the notes indicate what drugs and dose the patient was taking on admission?				
B. DOCUMENTATION OF THE ILLNESS				
i Were the initial medical notes adequate?				
ii Were the clinical problems clearly set out?				
iii Was the subsequent course of the illness well documented?				
iv Were the notes dated?				
v Were the notes signed/initialled?				
C. PATIENT AWARENESS				

i Is it clear from the notes what discussion took place
   and what information was given to a) patient ....
                              b) relatives				

ii Is it clear whether the GP was aware of the referral?				
iii . . . whether the consultant was aware of the referral?				

	YES	NO	N/A not apply	INAD inadequate
D. DISCHARGE				
i Physician's letter				
Was a letter sent? .... (days after discharge ....)........				
Does it contain adequate information about:				
a Diagnosis?				
b Discharge medication... (i/c total amounts given)				
c Patient information?				
d Follow-up arrangements?				
e Request for domiciliary support services, if appropriate?				
E. DEATH				
i Physician's letter				
Was a letter sent? ...(days after death ....).GP .... (days after death) ....).CONS				
Do they contain adequate information about:				
a Date of death?				
b Any associated problems?				
c Bereavement needs?				

GENERAL COMMENTS

_____

_____

_____

_____

_____

_____

Appendix E: Documentation Standard

(*see* Chapter 7)

Introduction

Laid out here are the standards for documentation of patients' notes in hospices; it is however to be accepted in such a multidisciplinary field of care, that certain information may be in the notes of other hospice staff. Each list has an introductory statement of standards.

General considerations

Standard: Medical notes should be designed, filled in and maintained to a level of intelligibility and access to information that is common to all units.

Audit criteria

- All handwriting should be legible.
- Entries should be initialled and dated by the writer.
- There should be logical structure and guide to any unit notes so a newcomer can find their way through them ie in an emergency; for audit; new in post; research; record search.
- Patients should have a unit number of code.

Cut off: Acceptable cut off:

Patient

Standard: There should be clear documentation of the patient's demographic and socio-economic background, and source of admission.

Audit criteria

- Full name.
- Address.
- Telephone number.
- Date of birth and age.
- Occupation (including prior to retirement).
- Where admitted from.
- Sex.
- Marital status.
- Ethnic origin.
- Religion.

Cut off: Acceptable cut off:

Next of kin/nearest relative/main carer

Standard: There should be a clear and adequate documentation about who is the patient's next of kin, the relationship and any special requirements they may have regarding communications.

Audit criteria

- Full name.
- Address.
- Telephone number (home and work).
- Relationship to patient.
- Special instructions with regard to contact.
- Similar details recorded for other involved relatives or carers.

Cut off: Acceptable cut off: (*NB* Some of this information may be in other hospice staff notes.)

Professional carers

Standard: The patient's relevant current and recent professional carers should be identified.

Audit criteria

- GP – name, address, telephone number.
- Consultants – name(s)
  – which hospital(s).
- Others – (eg social worker, Macmillan/support nurses, community nurses).

Cut off: Acceptable cut off: (*NB* Some of this information may be in other hospice staff notes.)

Referral details

Standard: It should be possible to identify the patient's main clinical diagnoses and problems as seen by the referrer, and the reasons why the referral was made should be documented.

Audit criteria

- Patient referred by.
- Diagnostic information.
- Reasons for referral.
- Date of referral.
- Particular problems.

Cut off: Acceptable cut off:

Patient's admission assessment – history

Standard: The history should be taken within 12 hours after admission and should be clearly documented according to accepted procedure for medical clerking; salient points about occupational disease and drug sensitivities should be highlighted.

Audit criteria

- By whom.
- When (date and time).
- Precipitating problems.
- Chronological order of medical events.
- Review of systems – bladder, bowels, weight etc.
- Family history, including health of carers.
- Social history including occupation (if industrial disease then onto cover of notes).
- History of allergies or drug reactions (also on cover of notes).
- What does the patient feel about their illness (where appropriate)?
- Patient's aims and expectations (where appropriate).
- Durgs being taken.

Cut off: Acceptable cut off:

Patient's admission assessment – examination

Standard: Relevant clinical findings at the time of admission should be documented.

Audit criteria

- Details well recorded.
- Orderly details of systems as examined.

Cut off: Acceptable cut off:

Summary

Standard: The initial medical assessment should be clearly and concisely summarized.

Audit criteria

- Problem list including diagnosis.
- Management plan.
- What has been said to patient/carers/relatives regarding diagnosis, present situation and future plans?

Cut off: Acceptable cut off:

Progress notes

Standard: The patient's clinical progress, investigations and important decisions or events during their stay should be recorded.

Audit criteria

- Clear.
- New decisions regarding management and important events documented at the time. These discussed with patient/carer/relative.
- A minimum of weekly note entries.
- Investigations requested with reasons.
- Results of abnormal investigations documented in the notes.
- Results of investigations filed in the notes.

Cut off: Acceptable cut off: (*NB* Some of this information may be found in other staff notes.)

Relative and carer support

Standard: The notes should contain adequate descriptions of discussions between staff and relatives or carers.

Audit criteria

- What have relatives/carers said (their opinions)?
- Relatives'/carers' aims and expectations.
- What have we said to relatives/carers?

- Documented in notes chronologically when relevant.
- Are there communication problems within the family – can we help/in what way can we help?

Cut off: Acceptable cut off: (*NB* Some of this information may be found in other staff notes.)

In the event of death

Standard: If the patient has died, the time and any special circumstances should be recorded; there should be clear documentation about notification of appropriate staff.

Audit criteria

- Time and date of death (burial/cremation).
- Who present (or informed).
- GP informed and when.
- Consultant informed.
- Bereavement follow-up considered.

Cut off: Acceptable cut off: (*NB* Some of this information may be found in other staff notes.)

Bereavement follow-up

Standard: If there has been special bereavement follow-up by the hospice unit, there should be adequate details of how this was carried out.

Audit criteria

- Documented (retrospectively) in the medical notes or elsewhere.
- What form and for how long.
- Any particular problems.

Cut off: Acceptable cut off: (*NB* Some of this information may be found in other staff notes, and the adequacy of this section will depend on how long since the patient died.)

In the event of discharge

Standard: If the patient was discharged, the notes should contain adequate documentation about drugs supplied and other relevant treatments, and what follow-up arrangements have been made.

Audit criteria

- Date of discharge.
- Letter to GP.
- Letter to consultants concerned (these letters should contain information: diagnosis, particular problems, discharge medication, what the patient knows and follow-up arrangements).
- Home care team alerted.
- Community agencies notified.
- TTO drugs supplied.
- Drug card or other documentation to patient/relative.
- Hospice day unit or out-patient attendance – if not what arrangements to keep in touch?
- Hospital consultant appointment made (if appropriate).

Cut off: Acceptable cut off: (*NB* Some of this information may be found in other staff notes.)

Appendix F: Final Form for Auditing Case Notes in Documentation Audit

(*See* Chapter 7)

Unit .... Auditor (Position/title) .... Date ....

		Not entered	
		But applicable	Inadequate entry
General considerations	Legible handwriting		
	Entries initialled/signed		
	Logical structure		
	Patient code or unit number		
Patient details	Full name and address		
	Telephone number, if exists		
	Date of birth		
	Occupations (present and previous)		
	Post code		
	Place admitted from		
	Sex		
	Marital status		
	Religion		
	Ethnic origin		
Next of kin/main carer	Full name and address		
	Telephone number, if exists		
	Relationship to patient		
	Special instructions with regard to contact		
	Same for other carers/relatives		
Professional carers	GP contact details		
	Consultant's contact details		
	Others (social worker, Macmillan, district nurse etc)		
Referral details	Who referred		
	Diagnosis		
	Reason for referral		
	Date of referral		
	Particular problems		
Admission assessment			
Examination	Well recorded		
	All systems examined		
	Relevant findings		
Summary	General state of patient		
	Plan of care		
	Note of what has been said to patient and carers		

| | | Not entered | |
		But applicable	Inadequate entry
History	Date, time and by whom		
	Precipitating problems		
	Present and past		
	Systems review		
	Family i/c carers		
	Social i/c occupational		
	Allergies		
	Current medication		
	Patient's views if appropriate		
Progress notes	Clear		
	Weekly at least		
	Reasons for tests if done		
	Results of relevant tests		
	Test results filed		
	New management etc noted at the time		
	Patient discussions noted		
Support relative carer	Notes of carers' comments		
	Carers' aims and expectations		
	Note of what said to carers		
	Note of any family communication problems		
After death	Time and date		
	Who present and informed		
	GP informed and when		
	Consultant informed?		
	Bereavement follow up?		
After discharge	Professional carers told?		
	Letter to GP and consultant?		
	TTO drugs given and details to the carer?		
	Arrangements for follow up		

Appendix G: Report on Documentation Audit for Sample Month

(*see* Chapter 7)

UNIT . . . FAITH

FILE No. 1
TOTAL SCORE (out of 11) 4
AREAS WITH MISSING DATA:

Patient details

        Occupation
        Sex and ethnic origin
        Religion

Next of kin/main carer

        Special instructions for contact
        Special instructions for other carers

Professional carers

        Others (social workers; Macmillan)

History

        Social, i/c occupational
        Allergies entered
        Pacemaker?
        Patient's views if appropriate

Progress notes

        Reasons for tests
        Results of abnormal tests
        Test results filed

Support relative/carer

        Notes of carers' comments
        Carers' aims and expectations
        What was said to carers
        Family communication problems

After discharge

        Professional carers told
        TTO drugs given and note to carer
        Arrange follow up

FILE No. 2
TOTAL SCORE (out of 11) 5
AREAS WITH MISSING DATA:

Patient details

      Occupation
      Sex and ethnic origin
      Religion

Next of kin/main carer

      Special instructions for contact
      Special instructions for other carers

History

      Social, i/c occupational
      Allergies entered
      Pacemaker?

Progress notes

      Reasons for tests
      Results of abnormal tests
      Test results filed
      Important events noted at time

Support relative/carer

      Notes of carers' comments
      Carers' aims and expectations
      What was said to carers
      Family communication problems

After discharge

      TTO drugs given and note to carer
      Arrange follow up

FILE No. 3
TOTAL SCORE (out of 11) 4
AREAS WITH MISSING DATA:
Patient details

      Occupation
      Place admitted from
      Sex and ethnic origin
      Marital status
      Religion

Next of kin/main carer

      Special instructions for contact
      Special instructions for other carers

Professional carers

      Others (social workers; Macmillan)

History

            Date, time and by whom
            Family (i/c carers)
            Social, i/c occupational
            Allergies entered
            Pacemaker?
            Current medication
            Patient's views if appropriate

Progress notes

            Reasons for tests
            Results of abnormal tests
            Test results filed

Support relative/carer

            Notes of carers' comments
            Carers' aims and expectations
            What was said to carers
            Family communication problems

After death

            Who present and informed
            GP informed and when
            Follow up note

FILE No. 4
TOTAL SCORE (out of 11) 5
AREAS WITH MISSING DATA:
Patient details

            Occupation
            Place admitted from
            Sex and ethnic origin

Next of kin/main carer

            Special instructions for contact

History

            Social, i/c occupational
            Allergies entered
            Pacemaker?
            Current medication
            Patient's views if appropriate

Progress notes

            Reasons for tests
            Results of abnormal tests
            Test results filed
            Important events noted at time

Support relative/carer

> Family communication problems

After discharge

> Arrange follow up

FILE No. 5
TOTAL SCORE (out of 11) 4
AREAS WITH MISSING DATA:
Patient details

> Occupation
> Place admitted from

Next of kin/main carer

> Special instructions for contact
> Special instructions for other carers

Professional carers

> Others (social workers; Macmillan)

History

> Social, i/c occupational
> Allergies entered
> Pacemaker?
> Patient's views if appropriate

Progress notes

> Reasons for tests
> Results of abnormal tests
> Test results filed
> Important events noted at time
> Patient discussions noted

Support relative/carer

> Carers' aims and expectations
> What was said to carers
> Family communication problems

After death

> Who present and informed
> Consultant informed
> Follow up note

FILE No. 6
TOTAL SCORE (out of 11) 5
AREAS WITH MISSING DATA:
Patient details

> Telephone number (if it exists)
> Occupation
> Sex and ethnic origin
> Marital status
> Religion

Next of kin/main carer

    Special instructions to other carers

Professional carers

    Consultant phone/address
    Others (social workers; Macmillan)

History

    Family (i/c carers)
    Social, i/c occupational
    Allergies entered
    Pacemaker?
    Current medication
    Patient's views if appropriate

Progress notes

    Clear progress notes
    Reasons for tests
    Results of abnormal tests
    Test results filed

After death

    Who present and informed
    Follow up note

TOTAL SCORE (OUT OF 66) = 27
PERCENTAGE OMISSIONS

Allergies entered	100%
Arrange follow up	50%
Carers' aims and expectations	66%
Clear progress notes	16%
Consultant phone/address	16%
Consultant informed	16%
Current medication	50%
Date, time and by whom	16%
Family (i/c carers)	33%
Family communication problems	83%
Follow up note	50%
GP informed and when	16%
Important events noted at time	50%
Marital status	33%
Notes of carers' comments	50%
Occupation	100%
Others (social worker; Macmillan)	66%
Pacemaker?	100%
Patient discussions noted	16%
Patient's views if appropriate	83%

Place admitted from	50%
Professional carers told	16%
Reasons for tests	100%
Religion	66%
Results of abnormal tests	100%
Sex and ethnic origin	83%
Social, i/c occupational	100%
Special instructions for other carers	83%
Special instructions for contact	83%
TTO drugs given and note to carer	33%
Telephone number (if it exists)	16%
Tests results filed	100%
What was said to carers	66%
Who present and informed	50%

Appendix H: Palliative Care Core Standard Statements

(*See* Chapter 9)

Standard no. 1 Collaboration with other agencies

Standard statement: There is effective collaboration with other agencies, professional and voluntary providing continuity of care and support for patients, and their carers.

Standard no. 2 Symptom control

Standard statement: All patients have their symptoms controlled to a degree that is acceptable to them, and achievable by multidisciplinary team intervention within current palliative care knowledge.

Standard no. 3 Patient/carer information

Standard statement: The patient and his carer/s have the information they seek, relating to the diagnosis and progress of the disease, care options, and allied support services available to enable them to make informed choices.

Standard no. 4 Emotional support

Standard statement: The patient and his carers have access, in confidence, to expertise in counselling, psychological and spiritual care, to provide emotional support.

Standard no. 5 Bereavement care and support

Standard statement: The carers of the dying person have access to bereavement counselling, information, and support services, including external agencies.

Standard no. 6 Specialist education for staff

Standard statement: Specialist knowledge gained through courses, work experience and seminars is kept up-to-date within the multidisciplinary team, and disseminated to other professionals.

Appendix I: Questionnaire used when Interviewing Patients in Support Team Care

(*See* Chapter 6)

We are working in several health districts trying to find out more about people's health problems and their need for health services. This survey will help in planning health services for the future.

We have contacted you because we are particularly interested in people who have had recent contact with the support team or with the hospital.

In this booklet there is a series of questions about any symptoms you have and any worries you or your family face. There are also questions about the services you are in contact with. Please answer as many questions as you can. Even if you are only able to complete a few questions the information will still be very useful.

The information you give is in *strictest confidence*. Your views and opinions will be recorded anonymously. The researchers who are interviewing people are Irene Higginson (a medical doctor) and Jan Lloyd (a nurse volunteer).

We would like to thank you *very much* for taking the time and trouble to help us in this survey.

1–3	8
4–7	9–10

BACKGROUND INFORMATION Date of survey......................

1. What is your age?...................................... 11
2. What is your occupation?...............................
3. When did you last have contact with: 12
   a) the support team?...................................... 13
   b) your family doctor?...................................
   c) your hospital doctor(s)?.............................. 14

The next section asks how you have been over the last week

Please answer referring to only the last week:

4. *Symptoms in the last week*

a) *PAIN*
   Have you had any pain?   Yes/No
   If NO please go on to section (c), if YES please continue

b) What effect did your pain have on you? Please ring one of
   the the following:

   0 = None
   1 = Occasional or grumbling single or few pains(aches).
       You are not bothered to be rid of the pain.
   2 = Moderate distress, occasional bad days.
   3 = Severe pain present often. Activities and concentration
       markedly affected by pain.
   4 = Severe and continuous overwhelming pain. Unable to
       think of anything else.

15

c) *Other symptoms*
   Have you had any other symptoms?   Yes/No
   If NO please go to question 5, if YES please continue

d) What was your main symptom (not including pain)?

e) Were there any other symptoms? If so what are they?

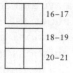
16–17

18–19

20–21

_____

f) What effect did these symptoms (not including any pain)
   have on you? Please ring one of the following.

   0 = None
   1 = Occasional or grumbling single or few symptom(s).
       You are not bothered to be rid of the symptom.
   2 = Moderate distress, occasional bad days.
   3 = Severe symptom(s) present often. Activities and
       concentration markedly affected by symptom(s).
   4 = Severe and continuous overwhelming symptom(s).
       Unable to think of anything else.

22

5. *Anxiety in the last week*

a) Have you had any anxiety or worries?   Yes/No
   If NO please go on to question 6. If YES please continue

b) What was the main cause for your anxiety? ....
   ....

c) Were there any other problems? If so what were these?
   ....

d) What effect did your anxiety have on you? Please ring one
   of the following.

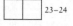
23–24

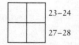
23–24

27–28

0 = None
1 = Worry over any changes. Not affected in any other way.
2 = Feel you are waiting for changes or problems to
   happen. This affects your concentration sometimes.
3 = Anxious often. Concentration markedly affected.
   Sometimes it makes you feel queer, gives you symptoms.
4 = Continuously preoccupied. It completely absorbs you,
   cannot think about anything else.

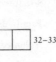

6. This question is about your *nearest family member or carer*,
please go on to question 7 if this does not apply to you.

a) Who is you nearest family member or carer? *Please ring*:
Is he/she your: wife/husband/daughter/son/sister/brother/
                friend/other relation/
                none of these: ....

b) What is his/her occupation? ....

Think about only the last week.

c) Do you think he/she had any anxiety or worries?   Yes/No.

If NO please go on to question 7, if YES please continue

d) What was the main cause for his her anxiety? ....
....

e) Were there any other problems? If so what were these? ......
....

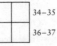

f) What effect did his/her anxiety have on him/her? Please
ring one of the following.

0 = None
1 = Worry over any changes. Not affected in any other way.
2 = He/she was waiting for changes or problems to happen.
   This affected his/her concentration sometimes.
3 = Anxious often. Concentration markedly affected.
   Sometimes it gave him/her symptoms.
4 = Continuously preoccupied. It completely absorbed
   him/her, could not think about anything else.

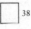

7. *Any time wasted in apppointments or tests*

a) In the last week do you feel you have wasted any time for
appointments or tests (or as an in-patient) at the hospital or
with your family doctor?   Yes/No

If NO please go on to question 8, if YES please continue

b) What was this for? ....

c) How much time did you waste? ....
Please ring one of the following.
0 = No time lost.
1 = 1–3 hours lost (eg trip for prescription which tired you).
2 = Half to one day wasted.
3 = One + day wasted.
4 = Two + days wasted.

8. *Are you able to get out?*

   Please ring one of the following.
   1 = on your own
   2 = with help
   3 = not at all

    41

9. *Who comes in to visit you and how often?*

a) Please detail below all the people including doctors, nurses,
   social workers, friends and family who visit you at home
   and how often they visit. You don't have to use their name,
   just say, for example, friend, family doctor, support team
   etc. The list below may help you.

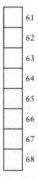

Person visiting .... Number of times per week or per month.	42	51
Relative	43	52
Friend	44	53
Nurse (other than support team)	45	54
Social worker (other than suppot team)	46	55
Family doctor	47	56
Volunteer	48	57
Member of the support team	49	58
Other	50	59

b) Is this enough? Is there anything else you would like?

c) Are there any practical aids or equipment which you think
   would help you or your family around the home, which
   you do not have?   60

10. *Communication*

a) Who has talked with you about your illness? Please tick below.

No-one has discussed illness	61
Family doctor	62
Support team	63
Hospital doctor	64
Hospital nurses	65
Your nearest relative/friend	66
Another family member	67
A friend	68
Other	

b) Who talked with you first? ....
   ....

   The next 2 questions ask about communication in the last week   69

c) *With the Support Team.* When you talked with the support team members in the last week how did you feel about the depth of information they gave to you and your family about anything you wanted to know. Please ring one of the below.

0 = Gave full information and you felt free to ask.

☐ 70

1 = Information given but not clearly understood. It confused you.

2 = Facts given on request, you would have liked more information.

3 = Evasive, avoided some questions.

4 = Avoided answering questions or visiting.

d) *With other Doctors and Nurses.* When you think of other doctors and nurses with whom you have talked in the last week how did you feel about the depth of information they gave to you and your family about anything you wanted to know. Please ring one of the following.

0 = Gave full information and you felt free to ask.

1 = Information given but not clearly understood. It confused you.

☐ 71

2 = Facts given on request, you would have liked more information.

3 = Evasive, avoided some questions.

4 = Avoided answering questions or visiting.

11. *Comments*

a) Do you have any comments about the hospital doctors or nurses?

☐ 72

b) Do you have any comments about your family doctor or the district nurses?

   i) Do you think your doctor is an easy person to talk to or not?

Easy	1
Not easy	2

   ii) Do you think your doctor has time to discuss things or not?

Has time	1
Not	2

   iii) Would you describe him/her as:-

Very understanding	1
Fairly understanding	2
Not very understanding	3
Or what	

iv) Altogether would you describe the care from your
family doctor as:

Excellent	1
Good	2
Fair	3
Or Poor	4
(No Care)	5

☐ 73

c) Do you have any comments about the support team?

i) Do you think the support team are easy to talk to or not?

Easy	1
Not easy	2

ii) Do you think they have time to discuss things or not?

Has time	1
Not	2

iii) Would you describe them as:-

Very understanding	1
Fairly understanding	2
Not very understanding	3
Or what	

iv) Altogther would you describe the care from the
support team as:-

Excellent	1
Good	2
Fair	3
or Poor	4
(No Care)	5

☐ 74

d) Do you think other people could be happy with the support
team?

☐ 75

e) Do you have any other comments?

Appendix J: Questionnaire used to Assess Staff's Views of Audit

(*See* Chapter 15)

The purpose of this questionnaire is to evaluate the staff's experience to the introduction and use of the STAS record.

1. What was your reaction to the introduction of audit in the palliative care units

   (a)   Good idea   ....
   (b)   Might be useful   ....
   (c)   Unsure   ....
   (d)   More work for the nurses   ....
   (e)   More paperwork   ....
   (f)   More change   ....
   (g)   Complicated   ....
   (h)   Of no use   ....
   (i)   Other comments...
          ....

2. Did you think that the introductory meetings were useful prior to its implementation?

                                        Yes. . . . No. . . .

   Please state reasons for answer...
   ....
   ....

3. Since the introduction of the audit do you find it useful?

                                        Yes. . . . No. . . .

   Please give reasons for your answer...
   ....
   ....

4. What do you find most useful about the use of audit on the palliative
   care units?
   (a)   Helps to identify problems   ....
   (b)   Helps to clarify problems   ....
   (c)   Helps to clarify what changes
         are taking place for
         (i) the patient   ....
         (ii) the family   ....
   (d)   Gives overview of patient's
         progress   ....
   (e)   Quick and easy to complete   ....
   (f)   Other comments...
         ....

5. What do you find least useful?
   (a)   Increased workload   ....
   (b)   Increased time   ....
   (c)   Another form to complete   ....
   (d)   Fails to show clear picture of
         patient   ....
   (e)   Not detailed enough   ....
   (f)   Other comments...
         ....
         ....

6. Do you think it is worthwhile continuing this method of audit?
                                          Yes. . . .   No. . . .
   Give reasons for your answer...
   ....

7. What modifications would you like to see being introduced?
   ....
   ....
   ....

8. Other comments...
   ....
   ....

Thank you for your co-operation in completing this questionnaire.

Index